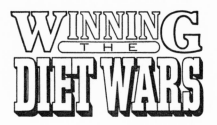

# WINNING THE DIET WARS

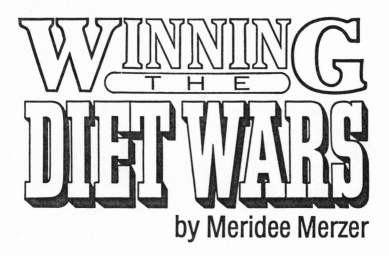

# WINNING THE DIET WARS

by Meridee Merzer

Harcourt Brace Jovanovich
New York and London

Requests for permission to make copies of
any part of the work should be mailed to:
Permissions, Harcourt Brace Jovanovich, Inc.
757 Third Avenue, New York, N.Y. 10017

Lyrics from "Junk Food Junkie"
by Larry Groce, copyright © 1976,
Peaceable Kingdom, Los Angeles,
California; used by permission.

Printed in the United States of America

Library of Congress Cataloging in Publication Data

Merzer, Meridee.
Winning the diet wars.
1. Reducing—Psychological aspects.
2. Reducing diets. 3. Obesity—Psychological
aspects. 4. Obesity—Social aspects.
I. Title.
RM222.2.M46    613.2'5    79-2765
ISBN 0-15-196378-9

Set in Linotype Times Roman
First edition

B C D E

This book is dedicated,
with affection and gratitude,
to my father and friend,
Dr. Philip S. Merzer

# Contents

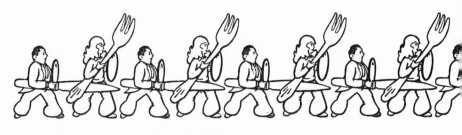

# 1 The Pursuit of Thin

Americans have more food to eat than any other people in the world—and more diets to keep them from eating it.

In the never-ending Pursuit of Thin, Americans have developed two opposing national pastimes—eating and not eating (dieting).

More than 40 percent of the United States population is overweight to some degree, according to the National Center for Health Statistics (NCHS). That means there are millions of people overeating every day. Consequently, there are millions of people who feel they're overweight and should be on diets. And, the NCHS reports, the average American does dutifully go on 2.4 diets each year.

The reason the average American keeps going on diets is simple: the weight doesn't stay off. The diets work only temporarily. The deeper, more stubborn weight problems remain.

The weight-loss problem is intensified because we live in a contradictory society. We glorify food, yet we abhor overweight. We favor a slender body shape for both men and women, yet we are food-obsessed, linking food to every sort of social occasion from weddings to wakes, from coffee klatches to corporate conferences.

We are trained from infancy to associate food and eating

with good feelings, such as comfort, love, well-being, and reward. Yet from childhood on, we are trained to idolize the slim and mock the overweight.

So it's no wonder that so many people spend their entire adult lives thinking about eating, veering from overeating binges to undereating on fad-diet regimes. This feast-or-famine syndrome has become a way of life in America—a self-perpetuating life-style.

Our diets almost inevitably fail. Why? Because people don't really understand the subconscious reasons they eat. Nor do they understand the underlying meanings that eating and food have in our culture. All most people know is that they can't become or stay thin. They are constantly engaged in the Pursuit of Thin.

But hardly anyone feels thin *enough*. Even top fashion models like Margaux Hemingway and Lauren Hutton—people who are highly paid just because they *are* so slim—find their lives centered around the continual Pursuit of Thin. "My whole life is a diet," Margaux Hemingway admits. And she is symptomatic of a culture that lives by the axiom "You can never be too rich or too thin."

The trouble is, for most people, no matter how long and how hard they persevere in the Pursuit of Thin, they fall short of their goals. Most Americans must ruefully admit, "Thin may be in, but fat is where it's at." And where is all that unwanted fat? Flabbily affixed to the hips, thighs, and stomachs of a whole nation.

Throughout their binges and deprivations, these people are valiantly though futilely engaged in the Pursuit of Thin. And all the while they're asking the same forlorn question, "Why aren't I thin?"

## THE FAT OF THE LAND

Despite the insistent Pursuit of Thin, Americans are losing the battle of the bulge. Instead of getting thinner, we are, on average, getting fatter and fatter.

2

According to the latest statistics from the NCHS, the average American woman stands 5 feet 3½ inches tall and weighs 143 pounds—15 to 30 pounds more than what the insurance companies' definitive "desirable weight" tables say she should weigh. That same NCHS survey revealed that the average American man stands 5 feet 9 inches tall and weighs 172 pounds—20 to 30 pounds more than the insurance tables' "desirable weights."

In the past ten years alone, the NCHS figures the average American male has gained four pounds. In the same period, despite a frantic search for an obesity cure-all, the average American woman has still managed to add on one more pound in weight.

Obesity remains a national epidemic. Supposedly, this country is caught up in a fitness craze—a new way of life based on physical fitness through running, jogging, and other sports. Supposedly, this country has also embarked on a new way of eating, deleting cholesterol-producing fats from the diet and adding fiber.

In principle, most people subscribe to the fitness craze; they agree with its methods and goals. In practice, the fitness craze is just that—little more than a fad. It has not made a major impact on people's daily lives. It has not caused most Americans to substantially change their life-styles in a direction that would cause permanent weight loss.

A 1979 survey conducted by the research firm of Yankelovich, Skelly and White, Inc., showed that most American families considered overweight a "serious health menace." Yet one-third of all families surveyed had at least one overweight member. Exercises for physical fitness were considered "beneficial" by the people surveyed. Yet two-thirds of the adults admitted that watching television was their favorite physical "activity."

Clearly, then, increasing awareness of the need for physical fitness isn't having much of an effect on the U.S. obesity epidemic. What *is* having an effect—an effect of weight gain—is the typical American diet.

## FAST FOOD, JUNK FOOD, AND THE HORN OF PLENTY

Americans are the world's champions when it comes to gobbling down calories. According to a recent study by the National Research Council, the average daily food intake in the United States totals a whopping 3,210 calories. Compare this amount to 2,940 calories per day in West Germany; 2,620 calories per day in China; 1,940 calories per day in India; down to a paltry 1,870 calories per day in Algeria.

How many calories do you actually need to live healthily and maintain your correct weight? About 2,000 calories per day for women and 2,400 calories per day for men. Adolescents and pregnant women, of course, require more calories.

Not only do Americans consume excessive amounts of food, but we as a nation consume food chaotically. For many families, snacks have replaced regular meals as the principal means of consuming calories.

Much of our daily consumption consists of "empty calories"—foods that have little intrinsic worth as sources of minerals, vitamins, and other nutrients. We pop down sugared soft drinks, crunchy snack foods, gooey desserts, and highly sweetened ice creams as part of our life-style. And then we wonder why it's so hard to stick to a diet of unadulterated, unfried, unsugared foods.

To most of us, a healthful, low-calorie diet is literally a shock to the system. Our systems are used to junk foods. Consumption of fresh fruits and vegetables has declined almost 50 percent in the past twenty years, so that processed and prepared foods now account for most of the average American's food intake.

When we purchase foods, we don't do it in a sensible fashion, thinking about balancing the various food groups, planning to eat enough vitamins and minerals. Instead, 46.8 percent of all the food purchased in American supermarkets consists of "impulsive buys," unplanned purchases made on the spur of the moment. These results were obtained from a

1978 survey conducted by the DuPont Company and the Point-of-Purchase Advertising Institute of New York. That survey showed that high-temptation foods, such as candies, pastries, and sweets, are also high-impulse purchase items. In other words, people walk through a supermarket, intending to eat "properly," but succumb to high-calorie items as they wheel their carts up and down the food-filled aisles. How else can you explain that survey's statistics? They say that 73.5 percent of all candy and chewing gum is bought on impulse, as are 70 percent of cakes and pies, 69 percent of pastries, and 67.7 percent of snacks and gourmet foods.

Purchases like these give the American diet its peculiar high-calorie bulges. For instance, the average American consumes 125 pounds of fat every year, as well as 100 pounds of sugar, according to the U.S. government report *Dietary Goals for the United States*. Americans are scared to death of raising their cholesterol levels by consuming too many fats. Yet paradoxically, the American's diet contains more fat than any other diet in the world, except the Eskimo's and the Finn's. In fact, within the past sixty years, Americans have increased their consumption of fats by almost one-third, according to the U.S. Senate's Select Committee on Nutrition and Human Needs.

How do Americans manage to devour all these fats and sugars? Accounting for the yearly 100 pounds of sugar is easy. Sugar is a common additive to virtually every kind of packaged food. Excessive sugar consumption begins with the dextrose commonly found in baby formulas. Sugar lurks in many adult foods besides the obvious soft drinks, pastries, and candies. Consumers Union discovered that certain brands of ketchup contain a higher percentage of sugars (28.9 percent) than do certain flavors and brands of ice cream. Sugar hides in salad dressing, gelatin, dry cereals, cream substitutes, noodles, and TV dinners.

Increasingly too, Americans prefer to eat out. About two-thirds of the American public eat at least one meal per week in a restaurant or fast-food outlet, and the trend is for more and more meals to be eaten outside the home.

Fast-food outlets get a larger and larger share of the business of Americans who eat out. According to a Newspaper Advertising Bureau study, over half the entire U.S. population goes to McDonald's at least once each month, while about one-quarter of the nation's population goes to Burger King, Dairy Queen, or Kentucky Fried Chicken at least once a month. Fast foods are clearly part of the American way of life.

Unfortunately, fast-food meals are, by and large, high-fat and high-calorie. A meal at McDonald's consisting of a Big Mac hamburger, a bag of french fries, and a chocolate milk shake adds up to a plump-producing 1,090 calories! And a Kentucky Fried Chicken three-piece dinner (three pieces of fried chicken, coleslaw, small roll, and mashed potatoes with gravy) comes to a hefty 830 calories. You'd be happier if you didn't even think about the fat and cholesterol content of most fast-food favorites.

Against such a formidably terrible national dietary pattern, a conventional diet—and dieter—stands a snowball's chance in hell.

## TURNING POUNDS INTO DOLLARS

Since overweight has become as common and as American as apple pie, an entire industry has sprung up to serve the needs of dieters. The diet industry is a growth industry in every sense of the word. Overall diet-industry sales in 1978 were estimated at $12 billion, with projected growth for future years pegged at 15 to 20 percent annually. NBC News has stated that $4 billion a year is spent on diet aids, diet pills, and supplemental vitamins alone.

Hofstra University sociologist Natalie Allon figures that Americans spend over $15 million each year on weight-watching clubs and clinics. Additionally, Dr. Allon estimates that we spend over $220 million yearly on reducing salons and health spas, over $100 million on exercise equipment, and in excess of $1 *billion* each year on diet foods, books, and literature.

As you can see, the diet industry is busy turning excess

pounds into dollars. The get-thin-quick schemes advertised by the diet companies have spawned some amazing success claims. Examples:

"Lose 13 to 22 pounds or more without eating less food. . . . The secret is a key ingredient discovered by a Medical Doctor" (advertisement for a book on bran diets).

"You can QUIT being a Foodaholic. Now lose weight effortlessly" (advertisement for a reducing clinic that specializes in "dynamic conditioning").

"The Amazing Diet Secret of a Desperate Housewife" (advertisement for the desperate housewife's miracle weight-loss book).

"The Missing Reducing Link Discovered. . . . Lose up to 6 pounds of fat and fluid the Very First Weekend" (advertisement for mail-order diet pills).

And, for the carriage trade, "Weight control means more than . . . losing pounds. . . . Develop new skills to manage eating behavior" (advertisement for a reducing spa).

Diet foods have proliferated and obtained an increasing share of the market. There are diet salad dressings, diet puddings, diet TV dinners, diet soft drinks, diet chewing gum, diet candy bars, diet breads, diet pastries, diet tuna fish, diet canned peaches, diet cookies, diet margarine, diet cheese, even diet matzos.

The only trouble is that not all diet foods contain many fewer calories than regular foods available at lower prices. Some foods labeled "diet" or "dietetic" are actually for salt-restricted diets. Or that label might simply mean that the manufacturer used saccharin and other sugar substitutes as the sweetener.

Whether calorie bargains or not, diet foods are often priced higher than regular packaged, frozen, or canned foods. They are sold at a higher general markup (about 23 percent) than most other prepared foods. This helps to increase their manufacturers' profits.

Weight Watchers International, the parent corporation for the Weight Watchers club franchises, was acquired by H. J. Heinz Foods, Inc., in 1978 for over $71 million in

7

cash. That's the same Heinz as in the ketchup and the fifty-seven varieties of beans. The reason Heinz found Weight Watchers so desirable an acquisition was not just the profitable Weight Watchers weight-loss clubs but the Weight Watchers line of food products—everything from frozen dinners and skimmed milk to an ersatz ice cream called a "frozen dietary dessert."

Speaking of Weight Watchers, it has become one of the most popular ways to lose weight in America, with over 12 million people having participated in Weight Watchers "classes" since its founding. An estimated 500,000 people attend weekly Weight Watchers "classes," where they are weighed in, exchange stories of caloric temptation and triumph, are exhorted by a "lecturer" on new weight-loss techniques, and applaud one another's announced weight losses for the week.

The parent Weight Watchers International corporation has a system of Weight Watchers franchises in the United States and twenty-six foreign countries, so weekly "class" fees vary, according to the particular Weight Watchers' franchisee's rate structure. Typically, an initial $3 to $6 registration fee is charged, followed by a fee of $2 to $4 per week for "classes."

But does Weight Watchers work? Do *any* of the diet industry's diet club or peer-pressure dieting groups—like TOPS, Diet Workshop, Diet Watchers, Calorie Counters—really work?

Very few statistics are available. Weight Watchers International does not release *any* statistics about their members' weight loss. They do not tell how many pounds the average member loses, nor how long these pounds are kept off. Why such secrecy?

One diet club, Diet Workshop, did issue the results of one study of its members. Diet Workshop functions basically on the Weight Watchers model but introduced behavior-modification techniques earlier than most other diet groups. According to a Diet Workshop study of about 125 women who had been "successful" in their program, 29 percent had maintained their weight loss for one year. That means 71 percent of the "successful" dieters on this program had gained back the weight they had lost within one year's time. This rate of success or failure is misleading, however, since most recidivism (gain-back) statistics are considered valid only after two years have passed, not one. The statistics on recidivism by even "successful" dieters are pretty grim. About 90 percent of all U.S. dieters who lose ten pounds or more gain it back within two years.

Some programs have been significantly more successful than others. The behavior-modification/weight-loss program at the University of Pennsylvania Medical School is widely considered the most effective in the country. Its recidivism rate is about 70 percent. That means about 30 percent of its dieters keep the weight off for at least two years,

However, the University of Pennsylvania behavior modification program is not typical of all or even most medically supervised weight-loss programs. Even if you diet under a doctor's supervision, you won't have substantially better odds than if you dieted on your own. Why is this so? Because the medical profession has been singularly old-fashioned and rigid in its treatment of obesity.

*THE MEDICAL MUDDLE*

The American Medical Association has announced its position on physicians' roles in weight reduction. An AMA spokesperson explained that the association "does not recognize any 'obesity' or 'reducing' specialty. Nor does overweight require a 'special' type of physician. Obesity should always be treated by a doctor as part of the patient's general health program."

This position seems logical, but it fails dismally in practice. Most internists, family doctors, or general practitioners simply do not have the time to work out the nutritional and psychological aspects of a comprehensive weight-loss and maintenance program with each overweight patient.

Lack of time is not the only factor that makes physician-guided diets so failure-prone. Most physicians simply do

9

not have very much training in nutrition and no training whatsover in obesity control. Medical school curricula are at fault here. Hardly any time is spent studying nutrition in medical schools; what little time *is* spent typically focuses on the chemical constitution of vitamins and the like. This does not then confer upon physicians a godlike omniscience about matters of weight control.

Some doctors—both M.D.'s and O.D.'s (osteopaths)—have set themselves up in weight-control practices. These "diet doctors" are not practicing a genuine medical specialty, however. There is no residency program in obesity control. There is no examination given in any state of the United States to certify doctors in a diet specialty, unlike the examinations, residencies, and diplomas that qualify doctors as surgeons, dermatologists, or psychiatrists.

There *is* a voluntary association called the American Society of Bariatric Physicians. This is the organization many of the more reputable diet doctors have joined. But this society is *not* a regulatory group for practices or procedures in weight loss and obesity management. Nor can the American Society of Bariatric Physicians award diplomas in a specialty recognized by the American Medical Association. So a doctor could call himself a "bariatrician," yet have no actual training or expertise in the subject.

Many diet doctors are general practitioners; others have taken their residencies in specialties like surgery or gynecology. Frequently, these physicians turn to weight-control practices because their original specialty didn't prove profitable enough. As Dr. Barbara Edelstein, herself a diet doctor, wrote, these doctors range from "good to terrible."

The worst of the diet doctors are outright quacks, charlatans who inject their patients with useless drugs and hormones. They have been known to dispense amphetamines freely, which can lead to serious drug abuse. Some of these doctors barely examine a patient. They have a nurse weigh the patient and take a cursory blood-pressure reading. The diet doctor may personally hand the patient a Xeroxed starvation-diet sheet and a box of "rainbow pills" (varicolored amphetamines, diuretics, and tranquilizers), then briefly harangue the patient, trying to mobilize guilt and shame as motivations for keeping on the strict diet. The better sort of diet doctors spend more time with their patients. They may tailor a diet plan to a specific individual's needs and monitor blood pressure, blood sugar, and, of course, weight. However, few of even the "better" diet doctors really consider the psychological, social, and cultural dimensions of a patient's weight problem. They tend to divorce the patient's emotional state and cultural context from their mechanistic treatment of overweight. And this limited view of obesity management tends to defeat even their best intentions.

What is needed is a holistic approach to weight loss and weight maintenance. This means the *whole* person, in his or her whole environment, must be considered before overweight can be successfully dealt with. Most diet programs fail because they pay a lot of attention to the diet—but neglect to pay enough attention to the whole person who is the dieter and to the world in which that person must function.

Much more medical research into overweight is necessary before more effective treatments can be found. As it is, very little federal money is going into obesity research, despite the government's recognition that overweight is a national epidemic. And meanwhile, millions and millions of people are engaged in the fruitless, frustrating Pursuit of Thin.

## BUCKING THE ODDS AGAINST WEIGHT-LOSS SUCCESS

This book is designed to help you increase your chances of winning the weight-loss game. This book will tell you things about weight loss that your doctor never told you—probably because he didn't realize himself that these factors could be crucial in determining your overeating patterns and their solution.

One underlying theme in *Winning the Diet Wars* is the

11

concept of self-knowledge. In the case of weight control, that means a kind of *consciousness raising*. People must have their consciousnesses raised. They must understand that their eating and overeating habits are part of a larger whole, part of a social, cultural, media, and environmental network. This network interacts with the individual's own psychological and physical makeup and creates a unique weight problem—which requires a unique solution—for each dieter.

As you read *Winning the Diet Wars,* you're going to find out about the many hidden factors that comprise a holistic approach to weight control. This will help you help yourself to maximize your chances of success in keeping pounds off permanently.

You're also going to learn about body styles, shapes, and "ideal weights." This new information may persuade you that you'll never have to go on a diet again.

*Winning the Diet Wars* will point out to you the myriad components that add up to your personal weight problem:

1. You'll find out the ways of personalizing your weight-control programs to increase your success in getting and staying thinner.

2. You'll become aware of the cultural, social, and media elements that make you want to eat and overeat.

3. You'll understand the role that emotions, especially compulsions, play in making you overeat.

4. You'll realize that your (over)eating habits are not unusual or strange. You'll see that you are not alone in the ways you binge, starve, and generally overconsume calories.

5. You'll discover some new strategies that will help you want not to eat.

6. You'll learn the real nature of hunger, appetite, will-power, wantpower, and mindpower.

7. Best of all, you'll learn to feel better about yourself.

The whole process begins when you start to realize that overeating and dieting involve a way of life—not just a weigh of the scales.

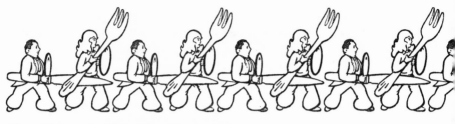

# 2 Food "Talks" to Us

Why is food so difficult to resist? Why does a chocolate cake seem to call out to some of us with a whisper that's more seductive than any lover's? Why do some people get turned on almost passionately to the charms of pot roast or fresh-baked bread? Why, in fact, does food have this great, irrational hold on us? Why does it cause us to break diets, to abandon good intentions of moderation, to eat when we're not hungry, to crave foods even when our bellies are full?

Why? Because food doesn't just sit there on a shelf. Food is constantly "talking" to us. Food sends out nonverbal "messages"—siren calls, aggressive shouts, seductive whispers, nagging groans. These messages often entice us to eat—and overeat. Some foods say, "I'm comforting" or "I'm exciting" or even "I'm Italian-American."

Food talks to us through the language of signs. As the young social science of semiology teaches, all inanimate facets of our culture, of every culture, give out "messages" or, as semiology experts call them, "signs." Food embodies many of these messages. It speaks to us directly, to our subconscious, to our implicit values and customary ways. It bypasses our logical thought processes and willpower and steers directly to that very vulnerable part of the mind—the sector of wantpower.

All these food messages serve as triggers that cause us to want food, often for seemingly irrational reasons. These eating triggers can also be termed "food cues." It is these food cues—their signs, their symbolism, their unspoken messages—that silently but powerfully stir up your appetite and your accustomed eating behavior patterns. Your body and mind are aroused to want food. You may already have eaten the food before you really know, on a logical level, what hit you.

You can detect the presence of hidden food messages when you hear catchphrases like these:

"I don't know why I ate that."

"I just felt I *had* to eat that—I needed it."

"Eating salad/bread/cake just seems 'right' now."

"I have this terrific craving for [take your pick] a Mars bar/a bagel/blueberry yogurt/chocolate-chip cookies."

All these actions, these desires, which seem to spring from nowhere for no reason, are simply our responses to the messages that food is sending us.

There are many ways to translate into clear concepts the silent messages food sends us. You can start by thinking of the different categories of food. Each of these food categories has come to mean something special and significant to us, depending upon our upbringing, our nationality, our social class.

What is food saying when it "talks" to you? What do vegetables "say" to you? How about fruits, meats, fish, bread, desserts, dairy products, soups? What does each of these food categories call up in your mind the minute you hear it mentioned? Those associations are a portion of the silent language of signs through which food talks to you. You "hear" each food "talking" to you, based on your past experiences, your likes and your dislikes.

Compare your reactions to other people's. For instance, each of the following food groups might suggest these associations to many people:

**Vegetables.** These might send out positive messages, saying, "I'm healthful. I'm cool. I'm elegantly simple." Or vegetables might transmit negative messages: "I'm rabbit food. I'm very good for you but often boring."

**Fruits.** They might say to you, "I hold sunshine inside me. I am a delicacy, a treat." Or they might say, "I'm a poor substitute for a really sweet, gooey dessert like vanilla fudge swirl ice cream."

**Meat.** This could say, "I'm full of strength, solidity, warmth." Or "I'm chock full of protein, so I won't make you fat." Or else, if you have a personal problem like a high cholesterol level, which might be aggravated by high-fat foods, the meat may speak to you in a different "accent," a distinctly different dialect: "I'm stuffed with saturated animal fats. I'll taste great when you eat me, but I'll kill you in the end with my high cholesterol count. Gotcha!"

**Fish.** "I'm protein-rich, but I'm less fattening than red meat. Hooray!" Or "I have a delicate flavor, appreciated most by refined taste buds." Or "I smell funny, and I never taste good unless you smother me with bread crumbs and eggs and gobs of spices."

**Bread and Other Baked Goods.** "I smell just like Grandma's kitchen with the delicious aroma of fresh-baked bread and cookies. When you eat me, you can remember the joy it was to be a well-loved child." Or "I'm very filling. I make you feel nicely stuffed inside, after you've eaten me." Or "No, no, don't come near me. I'll go straight to your hips and make you look fat."

Even a simple loaf of sliced bread or a humble doughnut can say many things to many people. But usually we don't hear the bread or the doughnut talking to us. We are so accustomed to their messages that they usually go right over our heads—and into our unconscious.

Think of food talking as analogous to radio waves beaming messages across the miles. The radio waves are present all the time. They pass through our buildings, through our cars, through our bodies—yet we don't see or hear them. We're not aware of their existence until we tune in to the special frequency of that transmitter's broadcast waves. But those radio waves have been there all the time, whether we're aware of them or not. The same is the case with the messages that foods—and other aspects of our daily lives that we take for granted—send to us. We are receiving, assimilating, and acting upon those messages, without ever consciously realizing what we're doing and why.

Now that you've become aware of some of the ways in which food can send out messages, you can delve more deeply into the actual language of food. These are the more complex messages that foods can carry. These messages can be conveyed by a supermarket full of products or by a single Twinkie.

The important thing is to become aware of these messages. If we don't listen to food when it talks to us, then we can never have an understanding of why we eat and over-eat. And then we can never understand the peculiar, almost inescapable way in which we are entrapped in the webs spun by food messages. These webs are emotional, social, and cultural in nature; their power over us results from the fact that food messages build up strength day after day, year after year, throughout our lives.

Food begins sending messages to us immediately after we're born. In fact, food is one of the few things that communicate clearly to a baby, even to a newborn. When a baby is given food, the language of food speaks out loud and clear: "I am nurture, caring, comfort, loving, warmth. I am Mother." From the infant's first sip of milk, the dialogue with food is initiated. And that dialogue never stops until the day we die.

Let's go through some of the most common messages that food sends to us. By hearing these complex, emotionally charged messages clearly, perhaps for the first time, you can begin to understand how tightly and in how many ways we are all held in the grip of food.

16

**Nurture.** One of the most powerful messages food sends out is "nurture." Nurture means nourishment. It means, literally, the sustenance of life. Without enough food, we would die. Or at the very least, feel deprived and uncomfortable. Because the nurture-nourishment message of food is so powerful, many of us associate the absence of food with impending doom, even with possible death by starvation. When you consider that food transmits the nurture message almost constantly from the first day of life, you may find it easier to understand why dieting (which is the absence of food in a society of abundance) seems so threatening, so depressing—even though we know it's good for us.

The nurture message of food is also closely linked to Mother and mother-love. It's obvious why this is so: in infancy, Mother provided nurture (food), and so Mother and food are immediately linked in our unconscious minds. Since the mother-child bond is fearsomely strong, even after the parent has died, even after the child has his or her own children, it's easy to see how intense and entrenched the nurture message of food remains throughout our lives.

**Comfort.** This message is closely linked to the way food talks to us about nurture and nourishment. The actual act of eating food is usually a pleasurable experience. The food has an agreeable taste. It feels good when it goes down the throat. The stomach feels comfortably heavy when the food eventually sinks down there. Clearly, food sends out strong messages of well-being and comfort.

Specific foods often carry very strong comfort messages. Let's say your mother always gave you chicken soup— "Jewish penicillin"—when you were ill as a child. Today, when you see chicken soup or think about chicken soup, it still says the same thing to you: "Eat me. I give comfort." Similarly, depending on your upbringing and life experiences, a beverage like warm milk, hot chocolate, or herb tea can say, "By drinking me, you can be good to yourself."

**Ethnic Identity.** The only cultural link many second-

and third-generation Americans retain with their ancestral homeland is through the stomach: kielbasa and pirogi for Poles; pasta and zeppole for Italians; challah and gefilte fish for Jews. Sometimes you even hear someone say, "I'm a stomach Swede" or "a stomach Lebanese." By this they simply mean that they're assimilated Americans, but they make a habit of eating and enjoying foods associated with their Swedish or Lebanese family heritage. If they gave up those special dishes in their everyday lives, they'd be severing ties with their roots.

That's why it might be excruciatingly difficult on an emotional level for a "stomach Swede" to give up lingonberry jam and Swedish meatballs when he goes on a diet. It would be just as difficult for a Lebanese-American to deprive himself of pita bread, pilaf, and honey-soaked pastries. These special foods that possess ethnic identification can speak to us very loudly and compellingly in their foreign accents.

Although foods may have a universal meaning of ethnic identification, the specific foods that say "Italian" or "Swiss" or "Brazilian" vary, of course, from culture to culture. In fact, foods that send out the message of "I am palatable" or "I taste great" can vary considerably from culture to culture. One culture's delicacy may be another culture's cause to vomit! Taking the American perspective, consider how repulsive you might find these alien delicacies if they were offered to you:

● roasted sheep's eyes (favored by North African Bedouins);

● the Malaysian treat of raw meat stuffed into bamboo shoots that have been carefully buried in the dirt and aged for two years;

● raw squid, tuna, and sea bass wrapped in seaweed and affixed to globs of rice (sushi, which is as much a national favorite in Japan as hot dogs are in America).

Similarly, good old American favorites like peanut-butter-and-jelly sandwiches on white bread or hot buttered corn on the cob might nauseate the Bedouins, Malaysians, and

Japanese. Actually, even the sophisticated French and Germans, whose cuisine isn't too alien to Americans, might be somewhat appalled by these all-American treats.

As the former president of the giant General Mills food conglomerate, James A. Sumner, noted, "The acceptance of foods depends on their fit in the existing cultural pattern. For instance, if you want to achieve acceptance in a society which regards fried grasshoppers as the ultimate in food elegance, then you must produce a product which looks and tastes and has the texture of fried grasshoppers." Clearly, then, local and national preferences and customs determine which foods are interpreted as tasting "good," as well as which foods will be imbued with ethnic identifications.

**Security.** Some foods create a sense of well-being; that is their message. They say to us, "Now that you've eaten me, you can feel secure and safe." For many people, a plateful of meat and potatoes conveys the security message most persuasively. Meat and potatoes are foods that have a certain bulk, warmth, and stability built into their physical nature. They fill us up, and that quality both enhances and conveys the message of security.

Hot foods generally send out the security message. Soups, stews, hot cereals, roasts, nourishing warm vegetables—all these foods say, "Eat me and feel secure. Eating me is almost as good as being tucked into the bosom of your family." Don't you feel safe, now that you're belching from your second helping of homemade stew?

Cold foods, on the other hand, don't usually send out security messages. Think about ice cream or cold cuts. These foods say many things, but they seldom say security or safety.

Still, you should realize that very few food messages are absolutes. These messages vary in meaning according to the era, the country, the social class, and the religious background of the people who hear the message subconsciously. All these factors can change the ways in which a certain food or food group speaks to us. Who knows, someday even a Good Humor bar may seem so traditional and old-fashioned that even that cold food (not now associated with comfort) will eventually say to people of some future age, "Eat me if you want to internalize security and safety."

**Reward.** This is one of the strongest associations food holds for many of us. From earliest childhood you have learned to consider certain foods—usually sweets and other desserts—as your reward for good behavior. The toddler gets a lollipop or ice cream to reward him for being good and not crying when he goes to the barber.

The school-age child is told, "You can't have your dessert until you finish all the vegetables on your plate." That's how most of us are indoctrinated into finishing everything on our plates whether we like it or not—a godawful habit to try to break when you've turned forty and are fighting an inflatable paunch.

As a child you finish your nasty-tasting broccoli or carrots, so that Mother will let you have a piece of spice cake with vanilla frosting. Or you bring home a particularly good report card. What's the parental response? Very often it's "Since you've made us so proud of you, we're taking you to the ice-cream parlor for a triple cone." Or the response could be "I'll make a batch of my special lemon crunch cookies—just for you."

After years of this kind of repetition, sweet foods, pastries, ice cream—all these addictive goodies—become inextricably linked in our minds with rewards for good behavior. As we grow up, we put away our childhood toys, but we take along our childhood attitudes toward food. We still hear certain foods telling us, "I'm your reward for being so good, for making your family proud of you."

Thus, the secretary gives herself an incentive to finish typing a long statistical report quickly: "Once I get done typing this, I'm going to take my coffee break. And today I'm even going to have a jelly doughnut. I deserve a reward for my hard work."

A sales manager celebrates each payday by taking his family out to dinner at a fine restaurant. He's using the gourmet-quality food as a reward for his labors and for "making the family proud of him," since he brings home a fat paycheck.

Unfortunately, when you associate food so strongly with the message of reward, you run the risk of bringing home not only a fat paycheck but a fat body as well. Many dieters succumb to the "food means reward" pitfall. They say to themselves, "If I keep on this loathsome diet all week long, then on Sunday I deserve to eat anything I want." *Deserve* is the key word here. The Sunday afternoon gorge is "earned" by the dieter having refrained from "good" food all week long.

"Good" food is, of course, not necessarily good for us. Usually it just tastes good to us, because we've come to associate cakes, pies, ice cream, fresh baked goods, starches, and such with reward. And so it tastes good to us because of the messages the food sends out, not because it's inherently scrumptious.

Certainly, this kind of once-a-week-I-deserve-it gorge satisfies the dieter on a deep emotional level. After all, we've learned to connect food with reward since infancy. However, when you're trying to stop overeating, it's not too logical to reward yourself with the foods that got you too plump in the first place.

**Affection and Love.** This is another of the very strongest messages that food can send out. When food says love, it's delivering this communiqué to your emotions in a manner that's very much related to nurture and reward. Again, the source of the message "Food is love, food is affection" has its origins in earliest childhood. "Mother loves me, so she feeds me" is the idea we have internalized.

This nurturing message transmitted by food gets generalized in later life. A wife wants to show her husband that she loves him very much. To give this message a tangible form, she might go out of her way to prepare a special dinner of his favorite foods. It's an adult extension of mother-love expressed in food.

Affection and love can be associated with purchasing and proffering special foods to the loved one. Richard was reared on southern cooking. It's difficult to find grits and greens, the food he grew up on, in the New England town where he and his wife now live. So, to demonstrate her love, Richard's wife drove fifty miles to the nearest big city to buy the southern-style ingredients Richard craved, so that she could offer him his boyhood favorites as a surprise. Richard's wife was using the food to "talk" for her. When she offered Richard grits and greens, she wasn't just giving him nourishment; she was letting the food say, "I love you, I care about you. You can see that by the time and effort I expended to find southern foods in deepest, darkest New Hampshire."

Another way food can say love very strongly is by the rarity of the food offered to the loved one. When someone important in your life offers you a delicacy (pâté de fois gras, Beluga caviar, even homey strawberry shortcake), you can sense that another message is being transmitted through the food. And that message is affection, caring, love.

Even a perfectly ordinary kind of food can speak of love very clearly, if that food holds special associations from your past. Colleen's grandmother would come to visit every other Sunday afternoon during Colleen's childhood. She would bring a chocolate layer cake with fudge frosting and chocolate filling between the layers. The grandmother brought this cake each fortnight as a silent message of love for her grandchildren. So it's no wonder that as a grown-up, Colleen buys bakery-fresh chocolate layer cake for her own children.

This is more than continuing a family tradition. To Colleen, even though she doesn't consciously realize it, purchasing chocolate layer cake means love for her children. It was a subliminal message the cake sent out to Colleen herself. And it is a message of love that Colleen's children have learned to hear and understand during their own growing-up years.

**Anger.** Food can also say hostile things to people. When Molly and Dennis have a furious argument, Molly "accidentally" burns Dennis's breakfast toast. When Dennis sees scorched toast on his plate, he would have to be deaf, dumb, and blind to the silent language of food not to realize the blackened slabs of bread meant hostility on Molly's part.

Withholding food is another way of making food say anger. Nick and his girl friend have just exchanged harsh words. Instead of taking her out for dinner, Nick "innocently" suggests that they skip the meal and go straight to the movies. He doesn't want to spend the money to take her out to dinner—in other words, he's withholding food. So Nick's girl friend could correctly interpret this lack of food as a sign of Nick's anger.

On the other hand, eating too much can be a sign of anger for some individuals. June has a lot of trouble expressing her anger openly. She knows that her anger works on a boomerang principle: June feels anger toward a person or an institution or a defective product, and she's unable to express that hostility openly. The anger boomerangs, and suddenly June finds that she's furious with herself. She has swallowed her anger, and that leads her to swallow food as well—masses and masses of food, a regular binge. June bites down on the food, and as she bites and chews, her mouth is silently expressing the anger that she cannot put into words.

Many people use food as a way of stifling and internalizing anger. They stuff food in their mouths so that they (literally) can't say mean things. Symbolically, they're shoving slices of bread down their gullets to keep down the words of fury that are bubbling up and threatening to pop out of their mouths. Thus, to some people, eating (and overeating) can be a symbolic way of saying, "I have my anger under control. The food is holding the anger down, inside me, so that it can't get out. Because if it did get out,

God knows what terrible things I might say and what terrible things might be done to me in retaliation for my anger."

**Belonging/Joining the Group.** Food is an integral part of the social ritual in all sorts of group events, from weddings to wakes. The next chapter tells in more detail how culture "talks" food. But here we'll limit ourselves to the way food says, "I belong here" or "I've joined your group."

Certain kinds of foods are meant to be shared and eaten by a group of people as symbols of unity and belonging. The most obvious examples are birthday and wedding cakes. If you go to a birthday party and refuse to take even a couple of bites of the birthday cake, you may very well be considered guilty of insulting behavior. Everybody else is eating the cake—like it or not—because eating the cake shows that they're part of the crowd, and, hence, a friend of the person whose celebration it is.

Food sends a strong message of belonging during the teenage years in particular. A favorite snack of adolescents is pizza. A pizza is meant to be eaten by a group of people. The very shape of a pizza carries the message of belonging and of joining a group: the pizza is circular and is divided into wedges. When you pull one wedge up, the gooey melted cheese stretches and sticks to the neighboring slices of the pie. Each slice, each person's portion, is connected to every other slice. The pizza is usually shared by two or more people, and any food that requires group consumption inherently carries with it a message of belonging and group unity. Therefore, it's not accidental that many adolescents go out for pizza with their friends—it's not just that pizza tastes good, but eating it symbolizes the unity of a friendship clique.

If we broaden the definition of food to include beverages, it's easy to see how beer and hard liquor are used as symbols of belonging. Gary never drank before he went away to college. During his freshman year, he found that all his fraternity brothers hung out at a campus tavern and downed pitcher after pitcher of cold beer. If Gary had refused to drink a mug of beer from a fraternity brother's pitcher, he might symbolically say, "I don't want to belong to your group. I'm not your friend." So Gary felt the subtle social pressure to share a beer and be one of the guys. Drinking the beer along with his frat brothers showed that Gary did, indeed, belong.

In more primitive cultures, certain dishes or classes of food are eaten only by members of certain groups, for instance, adult males. When a boy is initiated into manhood in certain West African cultures, he is allowed to eat "men's" millet dishes. When the boy eats these foods, which symbolize belonging to the adult male group, he is, in effect, announcing to the world that he's a grown man too, that he belongs to his tribe's grown-male category. Just like Gary and his fraternity rituals, the West African adolescent is eating a certain kind of food because it will make him "one of the guys."

**Power and Social Control.** Perfectly innocent food can be made to speak in accents of power and social control. It's not the food per se that exerts the power and social control; it's the way the food is used by other people—by authority figures.

The most obvious example of food used to signify power and social control is the way in which parents force obedience upon their children by making them clean their plates or eat foods that they find repugnant.

In this way, a limp stalk of asparagus can become a bludgeon—"You eat that asparagus because I say so. Now do what you're told." As the child dutifully forces down the asparagus, he's forming a series of negative associations with that vegetable. If that little tableau of his parents using food to exert power and authority is repeated often enough, the child will come to hate asparagus. As an adult he will harbor feelings of asparagus "saying" unkind things to him. A perfectly innocent green vegetable will then pack a wallop that the truck farmers never intended.

Food can talk to us about social control well past childhood and into adult life. Business executives may demonstrate power over their subordinates by making them eat certain foods at business lunches. Let's say Harry has a mild aversion to beef cooked rare. He goes out to lunch with his boss or with an important buyer. That authority figure has the opinion that beef just isn't beef unless it comes to the table dripping blood and nearly galloping off the plate. Harry tries to order his steak medium well done. "Nonsense," harumphs the boss or buyer. "You just try it rare. You haven't tasted steak unless you've had it rare." Harry may protest weakly, but he doesn't want to incur the authority figure's disapproval. So Harry will eat the steak rare. And for some time thereafter, when Harry sees a rare steak, his mind will be flooded with vague memories of being coerced, of having to do something he doesn't want to do. The food carries these memories for Harry, sending a message of coercion and power. Somebody else's power.

**Wealth and Plenty.** Elaborate and exotic foods on display at dinner parties can signal or reinforce the host's appearance of prosperity. Beef Wellington, pheasant with truffles, or Beluga caviar fairly scream wealth. When you're offered them at someone's home, you immediately get the message that the host is rolling in dough or else that he's appallingly nouveau riche.

Food has long been connected with wealth and plenty. One of the traditional symbols of prosperity is the cornucopia, brimming with fruits and vegetables. Since ancient times, such food displays have served to proclaim the condition of the host's finances.

Large quantities of plain foods can serve a similar function. It's the masses of food that speak in this case, not the specific food items. In the Arab world, for instance, a profusion of dishes must be served to guests in order to indicate the host's wealth and generosity. To say wealth to Arab minds (and mouths), the food must be not only of high quality but also served in superabundant quantities. Thus, the English expression "good food and plenty of it" is translated calorically into Arabic.

At diplomatic dinners and receptions, the food is usually of very high quality and present in giddy profusion, even at poor countries' wingdings. The message the overstuffed dinner plates and crammed buffet tables are meant to convey is this: "My country is rich and deserves respect." This message may operate in direct contradiction to the facts— that much of the world's population goes to bed hungry or even starving on any given day.

Rich food in delicately spiced sauces (that is, traditional French *haute cuisine* or classic Northern Italian cuisine) has long conveyed the message of wealth. Indeed, in traditional French *haute cuisine*, the general aim is to camouflage food artfully, so that nothing is instantly recognizable as a chicken or a duck. So if you can't figure out what your food is, but it tastes and looks as if it were prepared with expensive ingredients (butter, cognac, heavy cream, shallots, truffles), you may safely assume that the food is damned expensive.

**Status.** Since food can indicate wealth, it can also, obviously, indicate social status. Certain cuisines, such as the classic French style just mentioned, are sure indicators of status. These cuisines announce high status just as clearly as do Gucci leather goods, Aigner shoes, or Vuitton handbags. For both the traditional gourmet and the granola buff, the consumption (often conspicuous!) of certain kinds of food signals that they are somehow superior beings. They tell you their social, intellectual, or economic status merely by their food preferences.

For instance, a person who eats only organically grown fruits and vegetables, fertilized eggs, and stone-ground wheat bread *sans* preservatives, and shuns refined sugar like the plague, using only honey as a "natural" sweetener, is certainly emitting a lot of messages about himself. He's saying that he is a modern person, aware of his health, and rich enough to afford the rather elevated prices of most

27

health-food stores. In addition, this person is using his food to say that he's fairly anti-establishment, since organically grown foods and health foods have come to be associated with liberals or radicals. These are the connotations health foods carry *today*. As these foods grow more or less acceptable to the general population, they may send out quite different messages.

Similarly, a gourmand is using his food selections to say many specific things about his status. He picks a fine wine with an "insouciant" bouquet. He insists on *crème fraîche*, not merely American heavy cream. When he cooks, he uses shallots, not plebeian onions. The gourmand shuns fast-food restaurants (maybe that's wisdom, not just snobbery) and assiduously seeks out the very best restaurants—hang the cost.

With these food choices, the gourmand is using food to say many things about himself: that he favors traditional values, that he likes the best and feels he both deserves and can afford it, that he has more highly refined tastes and appetites than ordinary people. His food has said volumes about his status, even though the gourmand couldn't say a word about himself—his mouth was full at the time.

**Hospitality and Festivity.** In almost every culture, food is closely associated with both hospitality and festivities. A party isn't a party without some food. Even if it's just a few friends gathering together over a six-pack of beer, the host isn't considered hospitable if he doesn't throw in at least a bag of potato chips or a bowl of popcorn. By setting an ample table, you can say through the food that you really welcome and respect your guests.

Festivity can also be implied by the kinds of foods you set out. Party foods speak up clearly; they're different from everyday dishes. Perhaps it's the special effort that it takes to make traditional party dishes of your region or of your ancestors' nationality. A punch bowl says party. So does a plate of hors d'oeuvres. Even a humble bowl of onion dip can yell out, "Celebrate!"

28

Cakes are the most obvious examples of foods that say festivity. A wedding cake, with its curlicued and scrolled tiers, with its bride and groom figurines on top, carries the unmistakable message of celebration. Many cakes don't just embody a message but actually spell one out: "Happy Birthday," "Happy Anniversary," "Happy Mother's Day/Father's Day/Fourth of July." The presence of such foods is a vivid signal that we're supposed to party, to celebrate.

**Escape and Excitement.** Just as some foods tell us we're free to have a good time—*expected* to have a good time—other foods carry meanings of escape and excitement. It's usually foods that are strange or exotic to us that give us these messages.

Diane lives in a small town in Nebraska. For her, tacos or burritos seem strange and exotic. Therefore, when she eats these foods, she imbues them with a vague message of escape ("When I eat this burrito, I'm not in Nebraska for the few moments that those Mexican spices are on my lips") and excitement ("Well, these Mexican foods are so unusual. I wonder if they're as hot as I've heard. Will I need a whole glass of water to survive this experience?"). Of course, familiarity doesn't just breed contempt. It also takes the zing and escape/excitement factor out of formerly exotic dishes.

But for other people, strangeness isn't a prerequisite for food to say, "I'm exciting" or "I offer you escape to faraway places." These people use the act of eating as escape. As long as they're wolfing down food, they don't have to think about the problems of today. So Hilary might eat rather ordinary Rice-a-Roni for escape. The food itself isn't exotic, but when she's cramming the rice and vermicelli mixture down her throat, Hilary has a momentary respite from thinking about how she's going to balance the budget or from worrying where her son went when school let out two hours ago.

Thus, it's the act of eating and not the specific food that means escape to people like Hilary. Of course, if you can think *and* overeat at the same time, food isn't going to work very effectively as a means of emotional escape for you.

**Time.** Food is always giving off silent messages. It can even tell you what time of day it is, or what season of the year it is—roughly speaking.

Let's say you see all the people at a diner are eating pancakes, scrambled eggs with sausage, hot and cold cereals. You don't have to be a genius to tell the time of day by "reading" the foods' messages—it's morning, as indicated by the presence of breakfast-associated foods. If you were in Great Britain, the sight of small, thin bread-and-butter sandwiches, sandwiches filled with thin-sliced cucumber or watercress, or scones dripping with Devon clotted cream would indicate that it's late afternoon, because these are traditional tea-time foods.

It used to be that the sudden appearance of seasonal foods on market shelves and on dinner tables would indicate the season of the year. The first small new peas heralded the coming of spring. Blueberries and strawberries and cantaloupes told would-be eaters that summer had come. But nowadays, with the prevalence of freezing and the importation of formerly seasonal fruits and vegetables from warmer climes, it's nearly impossible to accurately tell the time of year merely by glancing at your dinner plate. Still, you can make a fair bet that watermelon says summertime to most people, just as a golden-brown roast turkey says Thanksgiving and a particularly elaborate baked ham says Easter.

**Formality and Informality.** Certain foods have very informal connotations, so when we see them, we think of casual get-togethers, of picnics and outdoor life. Other foods implicitly carry the message "If I'm present, you really should be wearing a suit and tie; this is a dress-up occasion."

You obviously wouldn't serve peanut-butter-and-jelly sandwiches at a formal reception. Peanut-butter-and-jelly sandwiches say informality. Or even that there are children present. Conversely, if you see a dessert going up in flames—

30

laboriously cajoled into an artful flambé—you can infer that the occasion is more formal. People just don't serve desserts flambé unless it's a special occasion. Otherwise, why waste all that expensive brandy to ignite a bunch of pears or peaches?

The way in which a food is prepared thus also signals informality. Steak served with a bearnaise sauce tells you it's a fairly formal occasion. Steak charcoal-broiled on an outdoor grill proclaims a family cookout, definitely informal.

The manners required to eat a food also speak a silent language. Foods eaten with the fingers (like fried chicken or french fries) usually mean informality, a casual atmosphere. Foods that must be eaten with a knife and fork speak with a certain degree of formality.

Of course, the languages of silverware or no silverware don't translate very well from culture to culture. In the Middle East and much of Africa, food is eaten with the fingers on formal, as well as informal, occasions. To lick the fingers and belch in appreciation of tasty food is also considered good manners and a sign of respect to the host in these societies. At the opposite end of the spectrum, the well-bred Englishwoman of a certain social class will use a knife and fork for virtually any food—even to the point of eating ice cream with a spoon and (ornamentally held) fork—as an indicator of simple good manners.

Aesthetics. The appearance of food also transmits many messages, quite apart from the food's cultural associations and emotional memories for the would-be eater. In many cuisines, the beauty of the prepared dish of food is just as important as the taste.

Food is designed to appeal to the eye as well as to the palate. A grayish slab of steak may taste perfectly decent and be highly nutritious. But since it's not sending off "beauty" messages, it probably won't taste too good to the eater who's aware of foods' aesthetic qualities. French cuisine is especially renowned for its emphasis on food that looks lovely, as well as tastes sublime. This is accomplished

31

with delicate sautéeing, with exquisitely colored sauces, with attractive arrangement of the various foods on the plate—balancing browns with greens, greens with yellows, yellows with reds.

The shapes of food also convey aesthetic messages. World-renowned photographers have captured the beautiful symmetry and tonal coloration communicated by perfectly ovoid brown eggs arranged in a wicker basket or by a flawless, un-bruised apple or pear reposing on an ecru china plate. They're following in the centuries-old tradition of the painters of still lifes, who recognized the beauty that radiates and speaks to us from Nature's works of art—fruits and vegetables.

**Religion and Spirituality.** Because many religions incorporate or forbid certain foods as part of their rituals and beliefs, food is rich in spiritual imagery. And that's why food can so often speak to us with holier-than-thou messages.

Food occupies a central role in many of the world's great religions (more about that in the next chapter, "Culture 'Talks' Food"). Just a glance at certain foods makes you instantly conscious of their religious or spiritual connotations. A holy wafer immediately signifies religious messages to communicants of the Roman Catholic, Greek Orthodox, Russian Orthodox, and other Christian churches. A sweet mixture of chopped nuts and apples bathed in cinnamon (called charoses) makes practicing Jews think of religion, because this food is used in the Passover religious ritual. In the Far East, a bowl of plain brown rice may send out messages about the asceticism and spiritual commitment of a Buddhist priest, who collects rice in his "begging bowl."

A devout Sunni Moslem expresses his deep-felt association of food with religion in this way: "We feel food is a blessing, part of one's spiritual values. There isn't anything more important than what you put in your body. That becomes an intimate part of you."

32

It's not just consumption of certain foods that's associated with religious and spiritual values and institutions. Abstinence from certain foods also communicates religious and spiritual belief systems. Thus, Mormons abstain from alcohol, coffee, and tea. Their religion forbids them to consume intoxicants and stimulants.

Observant Hindus shun beef. This religiously motivated abstinence from beef has led to the profusion in India of "sacred cows," which cannot be slaughtered for food. The sacred cows mystify most Westerners, who can't understand why reasonable people would deny themselves such a valuable food resource, especially in a country with chronic food shortages. If a practicing Hindu knowingly ate beef, he would be overcome by revulsion. The beef would taste foul to him, because his religious conditioning has made beef say horrible things to the Hindu's conscious and unconscious mind.

Orthodox Jews obey dietary laws that forbid eating shellfish (oysters, clams, shrimp, lobsters). Thus, to an orthodox Jew, shrimp says it is forbidden, that it is unclean, even that it is loathsome. But that message is perceived only by people whose religion conditions them to "hear" shrimp saying such things. To persons with different religious backgrounds, shrimp may say a lot of *nice* things: "I'm protein-rich, low in calories. I taste fresh and clean. I'm not too filling."

In other religions, proffering food to the gods may be used to obtain blessings, show respect to the deities, or propitiate demonic spirits. And, of course, Christianity makes much of the sacrament of communion, in which consuming the blood and body of Christ is seen as a symbol of blessedness. Food could scarcely speak in more devout tones than that.

**Generosity and Charity.** Since food is a staple of life, it's not surprising that gifts of food have long symbolized giving charity to the less fortunate. In medieval times, the lord and lady of the manor might donate food to the poor to show their Christian charity in tangible form. Since most serfs were living at bare subsistence level, the gifts of food had great meaning and were gratefully received.

In modern times, this custom of giving food as a form of charity has persisted. Churches regularly feed the poor, the aged, the sick. Politicians used to employ food as a way of symbolizing their generosity to constituents—and as a not-so-subtle way of binding the recipients' votes to the giver of the edible largess. The old-time politicos would send turkeys, hams, or baskets of food to their needy constituents at Christmas, Thanksgiving, and Easter. Those food baskets literally cried out the intended message of charity, generosity—and indebtedness.

More recently, groups like CARE in the United States and Oxfam in Great Britain have solicited food for the starving masses overseas. And so today the expression "a CARE package" has come to mean giving a gift of food for the sheer act of charity itself. Of course, when college students receive "CARE packages" from their families back home, the message isn't so much that of charity as of nurture and love. As always, the same food can have different meanings and messages, depending on the circumstances.

**Sex and Sensuality.** Sure, food can talk to us about altruism, religion, or status. But food also has a very distinctive voice that speaks of sex. There actually is such a thing as a sensuous calorie, because food can be used as a sex signal, as a sex substitute, as a sex enhancer (aphrodisiac), or as a source of sensual (as opposed to sexual) satisfaction.

One of the most erotic aspects of food is the way in which it's eaten. There's a sensuous feeling when certain foods touch the tongue and when they are swallowed.

Responsible scientists generally discount the notion of any food being a true aphrodisiac. But myths of sexually stimulating foods have circulated since ancient times. One of the earliest mentions of aphrodisiacs occurs in a medical papyrus of the Egyptian Middle Kingdom (roughly

2200 to 1700 B.C.). Even the Bible mentions aphrodisiacs in use at that time. And who could forget the carnality incarnate represented by Eve and her erotically charged apple? The ancient Greeks, Romans, East Indians, and Chinese all practiced the arts of culinary seduction.

The foods that have been thought to hold aphrodisiac qualities have varied from culture to culture, from era to era, but they have included such items as ginseng root, oysters, Spanish fly, and even the commonplace potato. In some times and places, sheer volume of food was considered an aid to lovemaking. As the Marquis de Sade once remarked, "A plenteous meal may produce voluptuous sensations."

The noted food writer Norman Douglas devoted a whole book, *Venus in the Kitchen,* to the cuisine of aphrodisiacs. And the great French gastronome Brillat-Savarin wrote in his classic *The Physiology of Taste* that fish held aphrodisiac powers, because they contained such "hot" or "inflammable" ingredients as phosphorus. Brillat-Savarin actually declared that truffles were "the food of love."

Even if food cannot actually serve as an aphrodisiac, the imagery of food holds a prominent place in loving and erotic conversation. In English, many words for food also have sexual connotations: cherry, lemon, wienie, honey pot, tart, nuts, tomato, dish, hot potatoes, love juice. The list is virtually endless.

Similarly, food words are used in English to signify affection: honey, honey bun, sugar, sweetheart, cookie, cupcake, dumpling, sweet pea, sweetie pie, lambie pie, babycakes. Or as the poet John Ciardi once joked about the Girl Scouts, "Remember, today's Brownie is tomorrow's cookie."

Food, language, and sex are intertwined from the most crass expressions to highly refined sentiments. And it's probably no wonder that we get overweight when food is constantly talking, calling, whispering, cajoling, muttering, chattering, or even guffawing to us. All this overly talkative food leads us right back to the perennial questions of "Why can't I stop eating so much?" and "Why aren't I thin?" Or to the corollary of those questions: "Why aren't I thin *enough?*"

Resisting the siren song of foods isn't easy. And it's made even more difficult when we realize that what we're up against when we try to control our weight is not just food talking to us, but also our culture "talking" food. And, as the next chapter shows, culture sure does have a big mouth.

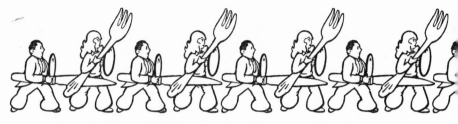

# 3 Culture "Talks" Food

Food may talk to us loudly and incessantly, but culture keeps up a pretty constant chatter about food, too. The ways in which culture "talks" food comprise the conditioning that every member of every society receives while growing up, in regard to food and eating habits. Your attitudes toward eating, overeating, dieting, and generally fighting the everlasting battle of the bulge all center around the ways in which you've been conditioned by your culture—by society, family, media, and peer groups—to think about food.

What do you consider tasty? What do you consider a great—though sinfully rich—snack? These tastes, these opinions about food, all originate not within yourself but within your cultural milieu, the context that influences every aspect of your life and behavior. And eating is just one of many behavior patterns that are culturally molded.

Unless the food is poisonous or in some other way injurious, there are very few absolutes or universals regarding what tastes "good" and what tastes "yecchy." For instance, natives of many regions of India favor snacks like ultrasweet banana chips or desserts like honeyed ghee (a kind of rendered butter) or even such exotic fare as sugar-crystallized rose petals. This is exactly the kind of food that would send most Westerners into a state of shock.

Conversely, the succulent steak and baked potato entrée is a standard item in the affluent American diet. But this highly favored American entrée would probably repel most good Hindus, who have been culturally trained from childhood to abominate the very idea of eating beef. Interestingly, McDonald's-style hamburger stands have opened in some large Indian cities. But instead of serving "all-beef patties, special sauce . . . on a sesame-seed bun," the Indian takeout restaurants make their hamburgers of pork, which Hindu consumers find culturally acceptable and far more palatable than beef.

It's not that people's taste buds differ from country to country, from culture to culture. It's that different cultures have taught their people that different kinds of food are appetizing or nauseating, delectable or forbidden. Why? For a variety of complex reasons having to do with local flora and fauna, with food scarcity and abundance. Thus, a Westerner would probably gag on grilled locusts, yet in certain parts of Africa, such cooked insects are considered a delicacy.

Culture talks to us so explicitly and in such detail about food and about (culturally) proper eating habits because food is so basic to every human being's survival. After all, food is a fundamental staple for the survival of all animals, including *Homo sapiens*. So it's no wonder that vast numbers of rituals and behaviors have developed worldwide, relating to how, when, and why we eat, overeat, or undereat.

Historically speaking, food can be regarded as one of the principal reasons for the development of civilization. Villages, towns, and, ultimately, cities sprang up in regions that were food-rich—rich in farm lands, in hunting lands, in fishing waters. Reading, writing, and arithmetic developed in the early Babylonian, Egyptian, and Phoenician civilizations to count and keep track of food supplies, to determine taxes on food materials, to render a permanent and accurate record of bartering and, later, selling for other goods and products. When you consider that food and its growing, gathering, and processing into edible form are central to human civilization, you can better understand why thoughts about food may preoccupy you for an absurdly large part of your day.

The way we record time and celebrate festivals is connected to astronomy. But it is also intimately connected to the growing and harvesting cycles. Most societies are organized around annual feasts, festivals, and rituals, many of which were based upon important times during the food-growing cycle. Even today, harvest festivals—replete with the display and consumption of lots and lots of food—take place in many advanced societies: Oktoberfest in Germany, Harvest Home in many European and New England farming communities, Thanksgiving in the United States. Other festivals served to commemorate planting times in the spring or the going forth of the fishermen in their boats.

The idea behind all these festivals was the celebration of nature's bounty, appeasement of the god(s), and a joyful recognition of the hard work required to wrest a more-than-subsistence living from the land and seas.

Culture talks food not only on special occasions and holidays but also in everyday life. Families get together over meals, particularly dinner. This is the time in which family members customarily share the day's happenings and solidify their feelings of family unity and family identity. In traditional societies, which are less harried and less urban, meals are intimately connected with the family group. To allow someone to eat a meal with the family implies some degree of accepting that person into the family's inner circle.

From biblical days onward, hospitality has usually been associated with feeding people, people who range from close relatives to complete strangers. Vestiges of the custom of using shared meals to symbolize familylike closeness remains with modern people. You eat meals with friends, not enemies. To intentionally seek out an enemy to share lunch or dinner is unthinkable. Why? Because underneath our civilized, modern veneer, we still associate shared food/ shared meals with family solidarity, with friendship's intimacies.

Whether at a business lunch, a dinner party, or merely at the table of an eating clique in a school cafeteria, the sharing of meals is still used to indicate a desire to be friendly or even familial. When we share meals with other people, we symbolically express the wish to initiate or maintain warm good feelings toward one another.

An out-of-town relative or old friend visits your city. The customary response: take him out to dinner or have him over to your own home for dinner.

You want to maintain a friendship? You and your friend and perhaps your spouses, too, make a date to meet for lunch, brunch, or dinner.

You want to sew up a big sale for your company? You take the buyer out for the much-derided but ubiquitous three-martini business lunch.

You want your family to size up and/or approve of a possible spouse? You invite him or her over "to have dinner with my mother." Such an invitation also indicates to your lover that the relationship is getting serious and may even culminate in marriage.

To use the jargon of the social scientists, the sharing of food is "a core experience." Sharing food (especially at structured, sit-down meals) strikes very close to most people's hearts and to their unconscious emotional responses. One sociological study in a prison showed that there were fewer violent incidents committed against guards by convicts when the guards and the prisoners ate their meals together than when prisoners and guards ate separately. Why was this? The sociologists claim the lowered rate of violence was due to the prisoners and the guards having shared "a core experience." Probably the convicts unconsciously still connected sharing food and mealtimes with friendship and family ties. When they shared meals with their guards, the prisoners unconsciously felt less hostility, because the guards were repeatedly in a social situation that the prisoners connected with friends and family.

Culture tells us from childhood onward that those people whom we share our meals with are the people we can trust, the people who are closest to us, the people we can depend on. The infant is fed by his mother and thus develops the deep, lifelong bonding that characterizes most mother-child relationships. As the child gets older and goes to school, he defines his friendships by the people he sits with in the school cafeteria and after-school snack shops. At the collegiate level, shared meals again serve to define friendships and cliques. The American fraternity-sorority system grew, in part, out of the "eating clubs" that are still perpetuated at the very oldest U.S. universities, such as Harvard and Princeton.

In adulthood, too, partaking of meals together (sharing food) continues to be a primary way of cementing friendships and business relationships. The junior executive who wants a promotion invites his boss home for dinner. The junior executive's wife will strive to serve an especially elaborate meal. Why? To symbolize her and her husband's high regard for the boss. If the dinner is a success, Mr. Bossman will probably look more kindly upon the junior executive. The boss will regard his underling more warmly, not for any logical reason, but for the primitive emotional responses that are generated by sharing food. That's a perfect example of the collision of culture talking food and food talking directly to us. The symbolic undertones and overtones of something as seemingly simple as a dinner party for the boss are staggering.

In some societies and countries, culture talks food even more directly. Most cultures are rich in words that describe foods and their flavors. China is a country that has, for centuries, been beset by frequent famines. That's one reason why the Chinese language reflects a deep concern for food and for getting enough to eat. The Chinese equivalent of the English "Hello, how are you?" translates literally as "Have you eaten today?" And the polite Chinese response is "Yes, I have eaten"—even if the respondent is half-starving.

In English we frequently use words that relate to food and eating to express emotions and to give color to our speech. For starters, just consider these familiar phrases:

- Variety is the spice of life.
- It's so easy, it's a piece of cake.
- The way to a man's heart is through his stomach.
- They go together like two peas in a pod.
- That actor is a terrible ham.
- He's a real cold fish.
- I'm fed up with swallowing your lies.
- You look good enough to eat.
- I hunger for your touch.
- Those egghead intellectuals are real turkeys.

The frequent, often imaginative use of food words to describe other aspects of our lives hasn't gone unnoticed by the social scientists. This linking of food and language helped inspire Fritz Perls, one of the founders of gestalt psychology, to base a philosophy of psychoanalysis on eating. Perls thought that it was no accident that we use the metaphors of food and eating to describe some of our most significant feelings, particularly feelings that deal with love and sex.

And the gestalt insights about food and eating have led to contemporary culture's solemn pronouncement "You are what you eat"—a statement that is likely to stick in the craw of any person who has a weight problem.

Since culture has repeatedly told us that food is so important, so vital to our physical and (particularly) to our social well-being, it follows logically that most of us experience dieting as an emotionally threatening act. Dieting is, after all, a life-style based on food deprivation.

And it's not merely the cutting down on food consumption that so disturbs us when we're on a diet. It's the fact that cutting down on food often means cutting down or straining social contacts. The dieter tells himself, "No, I can't join my friends for a big, heavy restaurant meal—I'm dieting." A mother or spouse might become offended because the dieter doesn't (over)eat to show how much he appreciates her cooking: "I sweated in that kitchen for hours to make your favorite dish, and if you're not going to eat it, I'll be very hurt." So the dieter can add guilt to the emotional consequences of the diet.

Not only does food have emotional and social meanings, but food and eating often carry religious meanings as well. Most of the world's major religions have some rituals or dogma relating to food. The Hindu proscription against beef-eating has already been mentioned. Certain high-caste Hindus also are not allowed to eat any form of animal flesh and are, in fact, required by their religion to practice strict vegetarianism.

Followers of Islam are forbidden to eat pork. Moslems also have ritual fast periods. For one month in the Islamic calendar, the month of Ramadan, practicing Moslems are enjoined against eating during the daylight hours. After sundown they are allowed to break their fast. The prohibition of eating (the ritual fast) concentrates attention, inadvertently, more on food and eating than ever. So it's not surprising that Moslem families have devised often sumptuous feasts for Ramadan nights, though the Ramadan days are food-free.

Many religions use abstention from eating as a means of ritual purification. Jews observe an annual holy fast day called Yom Kippur (literally, Day of Atonement), when they do not eat, in order to atone for the sins they have committed during the previous year. As with the Islamic Ramadan observance, ritual fasting on Yom Kippur and other Jewish fast days ironically often results in overeating on the day preceding the fast and on the day after, when special large meals are served *en famille*.

Of course, fasts are mentioned in the New Testament. One of the most notable instances of fasting is the forty-day fast that Jesus practiced while He was wandering and meditating in the desert. Jesus' forty-day fast became the model for the forty-day penitential and fasting period which

Christians call Lent. And until a few years ago, devout Roman Catholics had to fast one day a week by forgoing meat—the meatless or "fish" Fridays. In contrast, saints are commemorated in the Roman Catholic and Eastern Rite churches by special *feast* days.

Fasting occupies a prominent place in the practice of many Eastern religious faiths, notably Buddhism and Hinduism. The complete and partial fast are integral parts of the life-styles of the Buddhist monk, the Hindu yogi, and other Buddhist and Hindu mystics who seek enlightenment. Indeed, full or partial fasting for prolonged periods is one of the hallmarks of all religions' ascetics. And these ascetics have been respected, even venerated, throughout the centuries for their self-control and discipline.

In this way, culture has indoctrinated people via religion with the belief that successful fasting is linked to spiritual merit. Thus, when you break your diet, you feel guilty. Not just because you're staying fat, but also because you've assimilated the cultural-religious message that rigorous self-discipline in eating is connected to holiness, to a state of grace.

Religious dietary laws serve as powerful voices with which culture talks to us about food. The Jewish dietary laws are the best-known in this regard. These dietary laws (broadly termed "keeping kosher" or "keeping kashruth") are laced with food prohibitions: no shellfish, no pork, no ham, no bacon, no mixing of milk with meat products, even to the extent of keeping separate dishes and silverware for milk and meat meals.

During the eight-day religious holiday of Passover, traditionally observant Jews also abstain from bread and all baked goods that are made with yeast. Instead, they eat unleavened bread called matzos, which resemble large, ridged crackers. The matzos eaten during Passover recall the Israelites' flight from bondage in ancient Egypt with every bite that the faithful take. In this way, food is made to symbolize the history and cultural heritage of a whole people.

The Judeo-Christian culture we live in is filled with religious references to food. The land the Israelites were seeking was lauded as "the land of milk and honey"—that is, a place where food would be plentiful and there would be no hunger such as they had experienced in their slavery in Egypt. During their forty years of wandering in the desert, before reaching "the land of milk and honey," the Bible says the Lord fed the people with "manna from heaven."

Contradictorily, food is also linked with Original Sin in the Bible. Adam and Eve fell from grace when they ate the forbidden apple that grew in the Garden of Eden. The renowned French gastronome Brillat-Savarin mused about Adam and Eve's fall: "You first parents of the human race . . . who ruined yourselves for an apple, what might you not have done for a truffled turkey?"

The Christian ceremony of communion is central to many people's religious experience and observance. Communion derives directly from the Jewish observation of Passover. The Last Supper of Jesus and his disciples was, of course, a Passover Seder (a religious ceremony that is woven into a meal of symbolic foods). At the Last Supper, Jesus used the sanctified Passover wine and ritual matzos to allow his disciples to partake of his blood (the wine) and body (the matzo).

The later Roman Catholic doctrine of transubstantiation held that the wine and wafer (a direct descendant of Jesus' Passover matzo) were actually transformed into the blood and body of Christ when the faithful took communion. In this case, eating (the wafer) and drinking (the wine) are allied with a state of grace. This cultural-religious message conflicts with many other Christian messages that connect abstaining from food and drink with goodness and holiness.

Even if you're not Catholic, Anglican, or Eastern Orthodox, these values form part of the dominant cultural context in which you were raised and educated. They are part of your conditioning. Just as we have involuntary knee-jerk reactions, so do we have involuntary lip-smacking and swallowing reactions to food much of the time.

Another powerful way in which culture talks food is shown in the high regard we have for good cooking. Tasty cookery is one of the most important components of housekeeping. Not only does it take a lot of loving to make a house a home, it takes a lot of cooking, too. At the more rarefied gourmet and professional levels, cooking is transformed into a culinary art—an exquisite delight to both the eyes and the taste buds. This fascination with cooking is further transmitted when culture talks food through the printed word.

Cookbooks may not be great literature, but they sell well, year after year. Hundreds of cookbooks are published every year in the United States alone. Cookbooks range from those teaching basic American-style family cookery to those which divulge the mysteries of exotic foreign cuisines. Some cookbooks tout various health-food regimes, and others parlay technological advances into cookbook royalty dollars. Witness the flurry of "crockpot" cookbooks, published to exploit the recently invented electric slow cookers.

Culture also talks food in less permanent printed form. Most newspapers print recipes and food news, either on a daily basis or in fat weekly food sections, which are chocka-block with food ads and money-saving coupons to redeem on groceries. Even the casual reader of these sections is cajoled, seduced, and otherwise persuaded to add a new dimension to his life by eating some new type of food— whether it's instant stuffing or chocolate-flavored cold cereal or a "time-saver" product like frozen vegetables in boilable bags. Most of these products are nonessentials at best, potentially harmful and nutritionally empty at worst. But they are brought into sharp focus in the newspaper readers' minds by the onslaught of advertising.

Newspaper reportage on foods goes far beyond simply printing recipes. Often the paper's food editor will even offer suggested weekly dinner menus as a kind of public service for readers' families. Reportage extends beyond the newest food fads to full-blown descriptions of the latest fad diet—

the diet that's *really* supposed to work after all else has failed.

In glossy magazines, culture talks food in a nonstop gabble. Such magazines as *Gourmet, Bon Appetit,* and *Cuisine* are completely devoted to food, both the home-prepared and restaurant varieties. Other magazines such as *Weight Watchers* are obsessed with food in quite another way, advising dieters on how to eat while avoiding excess calories. It's symptomatic of this society's food obsession that even a magazine like *Weight Watchers* (ostensibly dedicated to taking pounds off) regularly features many recipes, plus pages and pages of advertisements for "legal" foods that dieters on the Weight Watchers program can eat without breaking their diets.

The American women's magazines—and their counterparts published throughout Europe, North and South America, Japan, and Australia—are notoriously food-obsessed. Many magazines like *Family Circle, Woman's Day, Ladies' Home Journal, Redbook,* and *McCall's* abound with ads from the food industry. The total advertising budget of that industry for 1978 was estimated at over $6 billion—and that buys a lot of full-page ads and TV time.

Like the American society at large, these women's magazines are torn between the desire for slenderness and the rampant desire of most people to eat, eat, eat. That's why it's ironic but not terribly unexpected when *Family Circle* sports a cover composed of a mouth-watering color photograph of a panorama of showy desserts—gooey pies, sweet cakes, frothy mousses. Then *Family Circle* surmounts this caloric Valhalla with a boldface announcement of another feature within the magazine—a fabulous new diet plan.

Thus, culture—"speaking" via the printed page—reflects the schizoid attitude we hold toward food. On the one hand, culture says food and eating are among the most attractive and pleasurable aspects of our existence, integral components of the much-sought-after Good Life. And on the other hand, culture warns us that we'd better not enjoy food and eating *too* much, because chubby/plump/well-padded/robust/heavy body shapes are unacceptable nowadays, both culturally and fashionably. These contradictory messages about food cause many painful conflicts for people in this culture. To eat or not to eat—that's the question of the day.

Mass print media aren't the only purveyors of recipes and food information in our culture. Word of mouth is strong, too. Recipes are handed down from mother to daughter, within families, within friendship circles. The methods of concocting certain dishes sometimes turn into family secrets. And this process of passing down recipes, occasionally keeping recipes secret, only serves to reinforce the high value we place on food that is both tasty and attractive. After all, as a culture we *must* place an inordinately high value on food, if we devise secret, cherished recipes for everything from tuna casserole to turkey stuffing to spaghetti sauce.

Of course, the most pervasive (and often insidious) way in which culture talks food is via television advertising. TV commercials broadcast skillfully constructed messages about food—that this brand of soup creates a homey atmosphere; that another brand of soup is so easy to prepare that it liberates a working woman from kitchen drudgery; that a third brand of soup mix brings a hint of continental sophistication into your otherwise mundane meals. Television commercials can make foods seem sexy, exciting, comforting, loving, and just plain irresistible.

The food industry has devised numerous multimillion-dollar advertising campaigns to market its products by appealing to our basic emotional needs. Their advertising strategies could be called Temptation, Inc., because they've inextricably linked certain foods and eating with emotional needs, emotional states of mind. The food-advertising campaigns have capitalized on the many symbolic meanings that food can represent. (Just look back at Chapter 2 for a list of food messages that might apply to your own weak points.)

These advertising campaigns focus on one or more emotional triggers to encourage TV viewers to buy their products. Kentucky Fried Chicken disseminated a series of television commercials that emphasized the wholesomeness, the innate goodness, and the family orientation of their fast-food fried poultry: "It's so nice / Nice to feel / So good about a meal / So good about Kentucky Fried Chicken." These warm, wholesome connotations add appeal to the chicken, as well as help to allay the housewife's fears that by taking the family to a fast-food outlet she's somehow letting them down by serving inferior or "lazy" food.

In the beverage field, Pepsi-Cola scored massive sales for years by associating its advertising campaigns with youthful exhilaration. Scene after scene of exultant young people engaging in athletics, games, or "fun" activities were juxtaposed with messages to drink Pepsi. As the jingle went, "You've got a lot to live / And Pepsi's got a lot to give." After years of televised indoctrination, many people cannot even look at a Pepsi-Cola bottle without having subliminal feelings of youth and vibrance associated with a sugar-laden, tooth-rotting carbonated drink.

Wheaties breakfast cereal for years has made its sales thrive by linking the product to the concept "the breakfast of champions." The Wheaties television spots similarly focus on athletic achievers, all of whom, of course, eat tons of Wheaties and look fantastic, even in late middle age. The series of Wheaties commercials featuring Olympic decathlon gold medalist Bruce Jenner intercut shots of a highly muscled Jenner laboring fiercely in the Olympic competitions—pitchman as superstar athlete. Then the commercial makes a quick cut to the Bruce Jenner of today, still looking fabulous and chomping away at a bowlful of "the breakfast of champions." The link made clear to the viewer: Wheaties will help you become not only athletic and fit but also a winner. In this success-oriented society, it's no wonder that a breakfast cereal that implies winning against stiff competition will become a perennially best-selling product.

Sara Lee, the trade name for a whole line of frozen pastries, has focused its television advertising on several major jingles, all very catchy and hummable, all keyed into satisfying emotional needs through eating their products. "Nobody doesn't like Sara Lee" went one jingle. This had a two-pronged indoctrination message. First, the housewife could buy a Sara Lee product and be certain it would please her whole family. Second, working on a more subliminal level, the "Nobody doesn't like Sara Lee" jingle functioned as a message that you *had* to like Sara Lee baked goods or else you weren't really normal, weren't really a regular guy.

A recent Sara Lee television advertising campaign masterfully zeroes in on the way food can symbolize love, both sexual and maternal. The video shots are a series of attractive young homemakers in gleaming, modern kitchen settings. Each homemaker sings a line of the Sara Lee jingle, which this time links a specific Sara Lee product to love. "I'm gonna poundcake-love my husband," one housewife sings sultrily, to impart a mild sexual innuendo to the commercial. The next, a wholesomely maternal type, croons, "Brownie-love my child." The ultimate message of the commercial—give love by feeding your family Sara Lee pastries, and they'll love you, too: "Sara Lee-love the ones you love / They'll Sara Lee-love you back." And that's one more convincing reason it's so hard for many shoppers to pass up Sara Lee products in the supermarket. Sure, the pastries are tasty. But the Sara Lee commercials' love message is devilishly compelling.

Temptation on this vast and ever-present media level works in two ways. It undermines the little willpower most compulsive/emotional eaters do possess. And, even more importantly, these industry-wide advertising policies create and perpetuate emotional attachments toward foods. Television advertising creates many of the subconscious attitudes the general public holds toward food and eating. The subconscious effect of the food industry's advertising crucially relates to the problem of weight loss and low-weight maintenance. Especially when you consider that social scientists estimate that 75 to 90 percent of all food decisions are made at the nonrational, subconscious level. Willpower stands very little chance against the wantpower generated by advertising, media, and the resultant social customs.

But these are just some of the effects that powerful media

advertising of food has on adults. The effect of food advertising on children is far more pervasive and makes for even more pronounced emotional attachments to food as these successive TV-watching generations grow up. Television advertising aimed at children has been under a critical barrage from parents' and consumers' groups for years. According to the Federal Trade Commission, $500 to $600 million of television advertising is geared toward children yearly.

Several consumer-action organizations have concentrated their ire over children-oriented TV advertising against the commercials for breakfast cereals, most of which are highly sugared. In 1977 alone, the breakfast-cereal industry spent $172.5 million on television advertising, much of it geared to children. The consumer-action organizations' objection to these commercials is that these processed cereals are highly sugared, low in nutrients, promote tooth decay, and tend to foster poor eating habits in children. The theory is that these poor childhood eating habits will extend into their adult lives and set the groundwork for a lifelong battle against a sweet tooth and against overweight.

One prominent advocacy organization, Action for Children's Television (ACT), commissioned a study of television food advertising aimed at child viewers. According to ACT's findings, two-thirds of those commercials were for "highly sugared products." Even more disturbing is the ACT statistic that children were exposed to seven thousand television commercials for sugared products every year. Yet during the nine-month period of the ACT study, children were exposed to a total of only four commercials for such nutritionally desirable foods as meat, vegetables, milk, and cheese.

The cumulative effects of this pro-sugar television exposure are bound to be devastating—and highly formulative of the child's lifelong attitudes toward foods. Some parents and teachers think that they can train their children to have better attitudes toward food, despite the prevalence of high-sugar and junk-food advertising on television. But even the U.S. Surgeon General, Dr. Julius Richmond, has stated that parents and school programs can't successfully compete with television advertising in teaching children about food and proper eating habits.

Thus, a child's eating and food-preference patterns are shaped more by the media than by parents. And these children will grow up to teach their own children—with a substantial assist from TV commercials.

However, long before print and broadcast media began chattering about food, folk culture and music started singing a food-eating song. Several nursery rhymes center around food images: "Georgie, porgie, pudding and pie" or "Little Miss Muffet sat on her tuffet, eating her curds and whey." Fairy tales also use food imagery prominently. Snow White falls into a sleeping trance because she eats a poisoned apple. Little Red Riding Hood almost gets eaten by the Big Bad Wolf. And why? Because she was bringing her sick grandmother a basketful of food. And just think of the trouble Goldilocks gets into with the three bears—all because her appetite got the better of her—"Who's been eating *my* porridge?"

Folk songs of every culture feature paeans to favorite foods. In the American tradition, several songs about food come immediately to mind: "Short'nin' Bread" and "Shoo-Fly Pie (and Apple Pan Dowdy)," which concludes with the heartfelt bottom line of a compulsive eater: "I never get enough of that wonderful stuff."

### ARTS "TALK" FOOD

Twentieth-century jazz, blues, and r&b songs have often used food imagery in their lyrics. Sometimes the food images have been somber and terrifying, as in jazz great Billie Holliday's "Strange Fruit," in which the "fruit" hanging from a tree was a black man who'd just been lynched by a white mob.

But most jazz and blues food-oriented lyrics haven't been about the fun of eating food but about the fun of "eating" your fellow human being. These songs made their food references blatantly sexual, such as "Candy Man" (sometimes called "Back Door Man" in other versions) and "Jelly Roll" (in which a pastry transmogrifies into a phallic object). The food-oriented lyrics in the blues haven't been coy. Often they've been straightforwardly lascivious, as in "I'm the spoon in her jelly" (to indicate sexual intercourse) or a man imploring his girl friend, "Squeeze my lemon, baby, 'til the juice runs down my leg." Obviously, the man in question is not discussing citrus fruits.

Tin Pan Alley latched onto food images in a variety of pop songs. "Honeycomb" was a big country-pop hit, in which a man described his incredibly sweet beloved as a human honeycomb. And then there was the saccharine, semi-idiotic lyric to Sammy Davis's big hit "The Candyman," who mixed his candy with love to improve the world. Not to forget a panoply of catchy ditties about love that won tremendous popularity, such as "Sugar, Sugar," "My Boy Lollipop," "Kisses Sweeter than Wine," "Lemon Tree," and the immortal "Yummy, Yummy, Yummy (I Got Love in My Tummy)."

Rock songwriters also incorporated food into many delectable tunes. Country-pop artist Jimmy Buffet wrote a playful ode to the all-American favorite, entitled "Cheeseburger in Paradise." Another food-related novelty hit, "Junk Food Junkie," catalogued the sinful delights of Pringle's potato chips, Dr. Pepper soft drinks, cellophane-wrapped Moon Pies, and the joys of mellowing out on a real junk food high. Joni Mitchell's artful "Chelsea Morning" captures a bowlful of oranges as its first image, then follows with the sun shining in "like butterscotch."

Ray Davies of the veteran English rock group the Kinks has written slyly satirical songs about our crazy love-hate relationship with food. In "Skin and Bones," Davies tells the sad tale of fat, flabby Annie who reduces herself down to emaciation: "She don't eat no carbohydrates, don't eat no buttered scones, stay away from carbohydrates, you can look like skin and bones." Davies himself can't seem to keep weight on, so he wrote a couple of songs, "Motorway

Food" and "Maximum Consumption," that lovingly detail the vast quantities of food he can devour while maintaining a rock star's skinny physique.

Of course, the food-symbolizing-sex tradition of the blues has also been adopted by the rock world. One obvious example is the hit single by the Rolling Stones called "Brown Sugar," in which the ultimate sweetness—the brown sugar of the singer's life—is reckoned to be the sexual favors of a young black girl.

The film world has also contributed some works that are based on the seemingly universal obsession with food and overeating. Gluttony is commemorated in such comedic cinema gems as *La Grande Bouffe* (in which the participants at a food orgy literally eat themselves to death) and *Who Is Killing the Great Chefs of Europe?* (another eat-yourself-to-death opus, which also offers a few satirical swipes at the fast-food industry).

In the theater, eating has offered playwrights a focus for their works. Thornton Wilder's *The Long Christmas Dinner* shows birth, life, and death, all encompassed within a family Christmas dinner that lasts for one hundred surreal years. In the comedy *The Play's the Thing* by Ferenc Molnar and P. G. Wodehouse, one of the central characters knowingly remarks, while downing an enormous meal, that audiences love nothing better than to watch actors eat onstage. In *The Transfiguration of Benno Blimpie* by the young American playwright Albert Innaurato, the main character, Benno, is a five-hundred-pounder who slobbers down food during the entire course of the play, so that he can achieve his goal—eating himself to death.

Culture reflects its preoccupation with food in many other ways as well. For centuries, artists have painted still lifes, in which fruits and sometimes vegetables have been rendered with painstaking detail. Photographers, too, have turned food into works of art. A famous example is Edward Weston's voluptuous photograph of a green pepper, which acquires a positively sensual appearance.

54

## DESIGN "TALKS" FOOD

Architecture is also used to express the importance that culture attaches to food preparation, consumption, and purchase. Take the care that is given to the design of restaurants. Elegant, expensive restaurants showcase fine food in beautiful settings, in order to make eating food a complete sensory experience.

Fast-food restaurants don't stress the Gracious Living elements of dining out, but their architects and designers have analyzed how surroundings encourage people to eat. Their studies showed that most people's appetites are depressed by the colors green and blue, but diners want to eat more when they're surrounded by reds, oranges, and yellows. That's why you'll see McDonald's and Burger King and Kentucky Fried Chicken establishments decorated in bright, warm reds, oranges, and yellows. It's not a haphazard choice, but a design developed to increase food purchase and consumption.

Take another cultural message that food is important in our lives—the typical suburban kitchen. This kitchen is lavished with thousands of dollars' worth of fixtures and appliances to keep food fresh (refrigerator), prepare food (ovens, ranges, food processors, toasters, meat grinders, electric frying pans, mixers, broilers), and to clean up the remnants of the food after it's been consumed (garbage disposal, trash compactor, dishwasher).

In most homes the kitchen is the center of family life. Meals are eaten there. A telephone is often installed there, and even a television, radio, and desk may be added, so that the kitchen serves as a centralized, multiple-use area. The kitchen is used more than any other room in the house, except perhaps the bathroom. Most family members at least pass through the kitchen in the morning, whether for a full breakfast or just a cup of coffee. The housewife centers much of her daytime housekeeping activities in the kitchen. She undoubtedly eats her lunch there, joined by any school-age children who happen to come home for their midday break. In the evening, the family members usually reconvene *en masse* in the kitchen for dinner and after-dinner chitchat and then return to the kitchen intermittently to forage for snacks during TV commercials. They may return to the kitchen before going to bed to get a glass of warm milk or cocoa or to wolf down yet another late-night snack.

The kitchen's significance is reinforced by the quality of appliances and furniture in it, as well as by its design (usually central to family areas of the house) and the care taken to make it attractive and emotionally warm. All these factors give off powerful cultural messages that the kitchen is important. And hence, food and eating are socially important, because they are so intimately associated with the kitchen.

Culture reflects its preoccupation with food in yet another way: the remarkable and often gargantuan forms that our food-purchasing places take. The American supermarket is a cultural artifact in itself—a monument to the American food industry and to the national preoccupation with eating. The very sight of the typical overstocked American supermarket is often enough to send some foreigners into a state of shock or bliss, depending on their previous cultural conditioning. There are acres of gleaming aisles full of cellophane-wrapped packages, colorfully boxed foods, fruits, vegetables, meats, fish, baked goods, toilet paper, pet foods, and floor wax. Recent refugees from Iron Curtain countries and from Southeast Asia have been quoted in newspapers as being stunned and overwhelmed by the cornucopia of foods and related goods in the typical American supermarket. This bemuses Americans, because we take all this excessiveness for granted.

These supermarkets function as retail shrines to the worship of food overconsumption. Consider that the average Jordanian villager of the 1960s could choose from only twenty basic food items in his local outdoor shopping bazaar. At that same time, the average American suburbanite could choose from over ten thousand food and food-related items in a well-stocked chain supermarket.

Just wheeling a cart down the aisles of a supermarket or even of a more humble urban grocery store is an exercise in temptation and self-control. It makes the ancient Greek gods' torture of Tantalus in Hades (starving, he continually reached for fruit that would forever evade his grasp) seem unimaginative by comparison. The supermarket shopper may scramble quickly past the cheese counter, past even the deli and bake shops, only to fall into a morass of irresistible temptation in the frozen-food cases, where frozen strawberry cheesecake, coconut cream pie, pizza, frozen yogurt, and a dozen flavors of ice cream are stacked alongside packages of sin-free foods like broccoli, corn, and slabs of rock-hard flounder, perch, and sole.

To negotiate your way through the twice-weekly supermarket shopping ritual without falling into some kind of food temptation (and hence into overeating) is to: (a) follow an incredibly tight budget with absolutely no money for nonessentials, or (b) qualify for immediate sainthood.

The American supermarket is not merely a place to buy food. It is a symbol of the entire American way of life—of the desire for possessions, the desire for superabundance, the desire to always have the best that money can buy.

Considering this national predilection toward food and eating, it's a wonder we aren't a nation of blimps, not just a nation of the somewhat paunchy. Culture talks food and eating to us so continually that it's hard *not* to overeat. What saves many of us from blimphood is the fact that culture talks thin almost as loudly as it talks food.

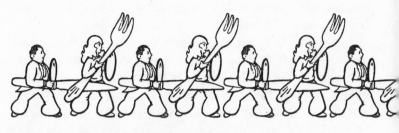

# 4 Culture "Talks" Thin

"Thin is in."

"You can never be too rich or too thin."

Those are the folk proverbs of our time. Other eras with other fixations gave us such wisdom as "A stitch in time saves nine" or "Sweet are the hands that do their own work." But in this age of diet consciousness and creeping obesity, our folk sayings are likely to be concerned with eating and thinness.

If King Arthur and his Knights of the Round Table were transported to this era and adopted contemporary concerns, they wouldn't be off on the Quest for the Holy Grail. No, far from it. Lancelot would be jogging and watching his cholesterol. Galahad would be playing tennis and going on the Scarsdale Diet. And Queen Guinevere would be sweating through Slimnastics exercises and girding herself for yet another go-round on the Quick Weight Loss Diet, the Atkins Diet, the Liquid Protein Diet, or the latest thing—the New Age Fasting Diet. Their quest wouldn't be for religious revelations but for perpetual slenderness.

The Pursuit of Thin is this era's and this culture's version of the Quest for the Holy Grail. And just as the Holy Grail proved elusive and virtually unattainable for King Arthur's knights, so too does the Pursuit of Thin seem a much-desired but almost impossible goal for today's general public to attain permanently.

But why do we engage in this endless Pursuit of Thin? Why are we willing to starve, deprive, humiliate, and torture ourselves to achieve "blessed" slimness? Because our culture places a tremendous premium on being thin. Symbolically, thin is good, thin is sexy, thin is healthy . . . virtuous . . . perfect. This culture has talked loudly and unceasingly about food to us. This culture has talked to us stridently and insistently about the joys of eating. But this culture, at the very same time, has also been whispering nonstop that being thin is the most desirable outcome of all.

How does culture talk thin to us? How does culture make us want to be thin—a desire that springs from deep, nearly subconscious roots? Part of our training about the desirability of thinness starts in childhood. Nearly all of us have been given parental, family, and peer-group pressure to get thin and stay that way. But where did our parents, our families, and our friends get those ideas? From media, from show business, from the medical profession, and from the fashion industry. These forces have combined to preach a cult of thinness, in which the jutting hipbone and the protruding rib cage have become "holy" objects, which we venerate.

Actually, the emphasis on super-thinness is a relatively recent development. The Pursuit of Thin is still not a universal phenomenon. In the Middle East and the Soviet Union, most notably, a plump or even portly physique is still considered attractive, perhaps even more desirable than slenderness. In the industrialized, affluent, and overfed Western nations, however, thinness is much sought after. In the West, the Pursuit of Thin began only in this century. And the serious Pursuit of Thin acquired its grueling marathon characteristics only after World War I.

In previous centuries, most people couldn't get *enough* to eat. Bare sustenance was the rule for most of the population. The heavier-set person was envied: he was rich enough to overeat. But industrialization and improved farming methods brought more and better food to the masses than ever before in history. The nineteenth-century scourge of tuberculosis—which brought wasting and emaciation to many sufferers—also helped to turn tastes *away* from slenderness in the last century. A very thin person might be vulnerable to or even infected with the dreaded and often fatal tuberculosis.

After World War I, several factors coincided to encourage slenderness. The military service had helped popularize the soldier's lean, streamlined physique. No place here for the previously fashionable embonpoint, the "banker's paunch." The fashion industry, too, turned itself into the quintessentially thin medium. Beginning with the flat-chested flapper look in the twenties—in which calves and even knees were exposed for the first time—women were persuaded to make their bodies less curvaceous, less rounded by feminine little poufs of fat or fleshiness. Instead, fashion leaders and designers urged women to look almost boyish.

At the same time, motion pictures were gaining in popularity. Films became a mass-entertainment pastime, with about the same importance in the average person's life that television holds today. The film medium, of course, adds weight to the person being photographed. By most estimates, a person will look ten pounds heavier on still or motion-picture film than in real life.

The film's leading men and ladies, consequently, had to be slimmer to look less awkward in the movies. A few pencil-thin actors and actresses like Katharine Hepburn, Greta Garbo, Henry Fonda, and James Stewart also helped to popularize the long, lean, fat-free look. Since films were creating popular idols on an unparalleled scale, it was only natural that average people tried to mimic the film stars, their popular icons. The masses tried, as best they could, to imitate the film stars' clothing, hair styles, and makeup. It was only a logical extension of this mimicry when the public soon tried to imitate the film stars' body shapes as well.

The film stars themselves eventually *had* to look like a

svelte breed apart from "ordinary" humanity. And the cinema idols, too, had to diet to maintain their seemingly natural slimness. The screen femme fatales of 1900 to 1920 were ludicrously chubby by current standards. But as the twenties wore on, thinness became fashionable with a vengeance. Few people today remember, but the young Greta Garbo was definitely fleshy, verging on *zaftig*, when she first came to America to make films. But the studio moguls insisted that Garbo shed the excess pounds. Suddenly, the chiseled beauty of her famous face was uncovered. And slenderness was once again reinforced in the minds of the public.

Meanwhile, the fashion industry—particularly the women's fashion industry—also did its best to ram the thin look down the public's throats. The Paris *haute couturiers* were the most influential in setting the new "thin" look. But that look was copied for American consumption in the factories of New York's garment district and eventually traveled to most Western-oriented countries. Many observers have suggested that the thin-look women's fashions that have predominated since the 1920s grew out of the conscious or unconscious desires of gay designers to make women look more like boys—hipless, breastless, with the boniness usually associated with extreme youth.

Many homosexual high-fashion designers were, wittingly or unwittingly, trying to make adult women look pseudo-masculine by eliminating natural female curves. This made fashionable women conform more closely to the gay male idea of sexual and physical desirability.

Of course, there have been influential women fashion designers, too. Some of the names that immediately come to mind are Chanel, Schiaparelli, Vionnet, Grès, Anne Klein, Mary Quant, Mollie Parnis, and Mary McFadden. But these women followed the male designers' lead, since they generally advocated the superthin look.

Large, pointy, uplifted bosoms did stage a minor resurgence in the fifties. This look was exemplified by the era's busty sex symbols (Marilyn Monroe, Jayne Mansfield,

Brigitte Bardot). However, the dominant trend in women's fashions has definitely steered toward a form of androgyny since the Roaring Twenties. Only in the sixties was this trend acknowledged, when the "unisex" look was openly proclaimed. And no matter how many sumptuous fabrics have been draped over women's bodies since the twenties, the underlying trend has steered steadily toward a form of unisex.

Until recently, women followed Parisian fashion dictates, even regarding such minutiae as whether hemlines were up or down half an inch this season. So it was no wonder that the *major* stylistic message—androgynously elegant thinness—came through loud and clear to the consumers. And the pattern for conformity to thinness was set.

Photographic and runway models were the human embodiments of the fashion designers' thin ideal. Models photographed in high-fashion magazines even today are almost impossibly long and lean. Hollow cheeks became stylish, and the protruding hipbone, devoid of voluptuously fleshy padding, grew to be much admired. At least by other women.

A survey of leading fashion models conducted by *Cosmopolitan* magazine showed that most of them weighed 110 pounds or less, even though they were predominantly 5 feet 8 inches to 5 feet 10½ inches tall. Cheryl Tiegs is perhaps the leading television and print fashion model of the late seventies and can easily be considered an ideal of contemporary standards of beauty. Tiegs weighs 120 pounds and stands 5 feet 10½ inches—and she is considered "full-bodied" by photographic modeling standards.

Women who see these high-fashion models in magazines such as *Vogue, Harper's Bazaar, Mademoiselle,* and *Glamour* get the implied message. Which is that they, too, must become superthin, supersvelte, in order to look attractive and desirable. This media-perpetuated ideal of thinness-equals-beauty sets off innumerable diets each year.

In the generations since thinness first came into vogue, many other factors have also coincided to help perpetuate the Pursuit of Thin. The models—both male and female—in print and television advertising are almost invariably thin. When a heavyset person appears in a commercial, he or she represents either a cuddly, parental prodding to buy the product (Mother Tums of the antacid commercials or Aunt Bluebell of Scott paper towels). Or else the heavyset figure is a villain, laughable or otherwise (like Mr. Cholesterol of the margarine commercials). Or else the plumper individual in the commercial is someone to laugh at (the squishy, rotund Pillsbury Doughboy; the chubby housewives who provoke smiles when they express wonderment over the efficacy of air fresheners or roach sprays). The attractive, desirable figures in almost any commercial are the thin people—thin housewives, thin he-man jocks, thin business-executive husbands, thin little kids.

The message comes across loud and clear to the viewers of print and television advertising: thin is best. The viewer's internal reasoning goes, "Everybody competent or happy on TV ads is thin, so I should be thin, too, if I want to be competent or happy."

The entertainment industry has followed the lead of advertising in the advocacy of thin. Romantic roles in theater, films, and television are almost exclusively assigned to thin actors and actresses. Entertainment programs make it appear that overweight people have no love lives, not even flirtations. Oh, heavier people do have a place in the entertainment media but usually as villains, servants, comedians, or the elderly. On television in particular, there is no room —or at least no casting—for anyone but the slender, with a few character actors as the oft-cited exceptions. When heavier people do appear on television, it's principally as stand-up comics on variety shows (Rodney Dangerfield and the late Totie Fields are notable examples) or as comedians on situation comedies (Jackie Gleason in "The.Honeymooners," Carroll O'Connor as Archie Bunker in "All in the Family").

Even the popular music field has been limited principally to thin performers in recent generations and thus has contributed to convincing the public that thin is the only way to be. In the days of radio, when the performer wasn't seen by the audience, a hefty songstress like Kate Smith could make herself into a widely beloved star. Today, however, the pop and rock stars serve to promulgate the ideal of slenderness to another generation of young people. Olivia Newton-John, Donna Summer, Peter Frampton, and Rod Stewart are typical slim-to-the-point-of-skinny role models from the pop music medium.

Rock stars in the sixties gave the skinny look a new credibility for men. Previously, muscular builds had been permissible, even preferred, for young American males. But with the rise of British rock groups, who were often semi-emaciated, young male fans began to identify with masculine idols who were too thin to sport muscles. It was hard for teenage boys, identifying with superslim idols like Mick Jagger or Led Zeppelin's Robert Plant, *not* to think that skinniness was preferable to even an average physique.

Besides, the clothes in style for young men in the heyday of the sixties rock idols *looked* much better on a skinny frame. Tight jeans, body shirts open halfway down the chest, and skimpy ribbed sweaters all looked better on very thin young men than on the more muscular and huskily built. The young men were learning the same fashion lesson that women had been indoctrinated with for decades: thin is in.

In fact, if you wanted to fit into stylish clothes, you had to be thin. Or else nothing fashionable would fit you. Women's clothing, of course, has gone through several phases in the past fifty years, in which extreme slenderness has been essential to the chic look. Sheath dresses and tightly cinched wasp waistlines did nothing to encourage overeating. If a woman gained even a couple of pounds, she might burst out of such clothes—literally. The miniskirt worked only if a grown woman could look like a little girl: toothpick legs and a smallish or flat bosom, so as not to break up the line of the minuscule dresses.

Looser clothing, a more free and relaxed way of dressing,

became fashionable a few years ago. But many designers predicted that the majority of American women would not go too far with the overblown shapes. These women had worked too hard maintaining slender bodies to let all that effort go to waste under the camouflage of yards and yards of billowy fabrics. So the sheath skirt made a comeback. Even more popular, however, were the straight-legged "cigarette" jeans and trousers for women.

These straight-leg pants were cut with such extreme narrowness that one doctor who specializes in treating anorexics (pathologically underweight people) said that no woman of normal weight could get her thigh into such a trouser leg without feeling she was too fat and had to lose some weight, pronto. This doctor claimed such narrowly cut but fashionable clothes helped drive some people into health-threatening diet marathons.

Of course, the medical profession has concurrently legitimized the ideal of thinness that was first set out by the fashion industry and by the media. Physicians aren't exempt from being influenced by the cultural bias in favor of thinness. As members of this society, doctors, too, have grown up with an enormous respect for thinness and a corresponding disrespect for heaviness. Most doctors, however, will deny that they, too, are influenced by cultural trends and fashion fads regarding slimness. The physicians usually explain that their abhorrence of overweight stems from the correlation of obesity with certain diseases.

Gross obesity has certainly been linked to heart disease and diabetes. Gross obesity has not been proved to cause the diseases, but the presence of obesity aggravates such conditions to potentially fatal levels. But mild obesity has *not* been shown to cause ill health. In fact, many weight-loss experts, such as Dr. Neil Solomon, say that the prevalent yo-yo syndrome (losing and regaining weight over and over again) may actually be more physiologically harmful than consistent mild overweight.

The medical profession's concepts of ideal weight and overweight derive in large part from the insurance industry's actuarial tables. The first major insurance studies that changed Americans' concept of the "healthy" weight to be were issued in 1912. The effects of the actuarial tables' ideal weights gradually percolated through the consciousness of the medical profession. Today's physicians have completely accepted the actuarial findings that linked overweight to disease and increased mortality. As physical anthropologist Anne Scott Beller puts it, these physicians have "mastered the official orthodoxy that fat is suicidal; a sin . . . at best; and at worst a sort of felony."

In 1959, the insurance industry published a new study that replaced the 1912 concept of average weights with "ideal weights." By comparing these actuarial "ideal weights" with the National Center for Health Statistics' figures, we discover that over 40 percent of the female adult population and nearly as high a percentage of the adult male population are considerably overweight by the "ideal weight" standards. That sounds fairly horrific, but the flabby American populace doesn't fare as badly as the West Germans. One study recently published by the Baden-Württemberg State Medical Association figures that the obesity rate for West German men and women runs to nearly 70 percent of the population!

The "ideal" or "desirable" weights listed in the actuarial tables have come under fire by many obesity experts. They have pointed out that these ideal-weight tables are not characteristic of the population as a whole but reflect mainly on the relatively affluent, prudent people who purchase insurance. Even fit, muscular people such as professional athletes (i.e., football players) are judged "fat" by these standards. Clearly, then, something is amiss. Still, the medical profession, by and large, has accepted the actuarial standards as the gospel truth. The doctors have been passing along these ideals of body weight to their patients. And thus, unrealistic concepts of fat and thin are further perpetuated.

Physicians aid culture in telling us that thin is great. "Most M.D.'s treat fat people with disrespect, contempt, insults, even sadism—they scream and carry on at people, because they don't lose weight," notes Dr. Theodore Isaac

Rubin, a psychiatrist who is a prominent weight-loss expert. Rubin cites an almost irrational prejudice toward super-thinness on the part of most physicians. Rubin believes, "Thinness is overvalued. Gross thinness, super-thinness, is as damaging to health as is gross obesity."

The very thin are subject to certain ailments, such as chronic infections, as compared to the grossly overweight people's tendency toward heart disease and diabetes. So unnatural thinness—the kind of thinness that must be maintained by constant, rigorous dieting—isn't necessarily good for you.

But this society has ignored any possible health hazards connected with super-thinness, because so many other cultural factors have worked to create a cult of beauty and desirability around being thin. Rubin and other weight-loss specialists have also cited a general medical ignorance about the psychological and cultural factors involved in weight loss, weight gain, and weight maintenance. "Most doctors aren't willing even to consider all the psychological ramifications of losing weight and keeping it off," Rubin says.

Still another factor that makes super-thinness seem desirable is the strong link we perceive between slenderness and youth. This is an extremely youth-oriented culture. Although the population's average age is steadily increasing, most people still want to give the illusion of being young. Youthfulness is associated with many positive attributes: beauty, trendiness, fitness, strength, virility. By linking thinness with youth, the Pursuit of Thin gains still more adherents.

But not every era has associated thinness with youth. The seventeenth-century English poet John Dryden wrote, "I am resolved to grow fat and look young till forty." This clearly reflects his century's association of fleshiness with youthfulness. In those days, old age was connected with scrawniness, gauntness, jutting bones. Today those same attributes are much admired and are considered sure signs of youthfulness (no matter what your actual age). This linkage of super-thinness with youth actually simulates the body build of a still-growing, gangly adolescent boy. It's another instance of the Pursuit of Thin being (partially) the pursuit of androgyny in disguise.

The overall message of our culture about thinness is that thinness is a kind of magic. Thinness is accredited with miraculous powers. Doctors tell us that thinness equals health and fitness and longevity. The fashion magazines tell us that thinness equals beauty and chic. The garment industry equates thinness with stylishness. The entertainment industry links thinness with romantic desirability and competence, even success.

Some folk wisdom of this culture holds that thinness goes along with sexual fulfillment. Thinness is also supposed to be intimately tied to energy, vivacity, self-discipline, self-mastery, popularity, advancement on the job. In short, being thin is supposed to make you happy. In truth, getting thin doesn't change the problems inherent in your personality or in your life situation. What getting thin does do is help you to conform to this culture's idea of what is attractive and acceptable.

Summing up: the message that culture "talks" about thin is that thin is magic. Thin will solve your problems. Thin will give you an edge on other people. Thin can make all things possible.

The only trouble is that for a lot of people, getting thin and staying that way are practically impossible.

One of the reasons it's so hard to get thin and stay that way is because of our unique eating personalities, our peculiar habits that surround the way we eat, the way we live with food.

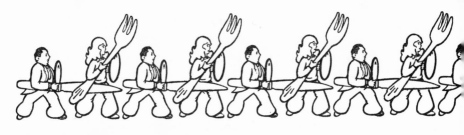

# 5  Emotions "Eat" Us

By now, you've examined some reasons why it's so hard to resist food. We are conditioned from infancy by our culture, society, and media to believe that food and eating constitute some of the great pleasures of life.

As the German philosopher Dr. Wilhelm Stekhel put it, "If there were no such thing as eating, we should have to invent it to save man from despairing." In other words, eating—and overeating—are the primary means by which many people manage to cope with life's traumas and with everyday anxieties and stresses.

We have already seen how food talks to us, how culture talks food. Now we can begin to focus on how we tend to eat and overeat when our emotions "eat" us. The self-help organization Overeaters Anonymous has a catchphrase: "It wasn't what I was eating; it was what was eating me." This is how Overeaters Anonymous expresses the very real emotional component that is present in so much of our overeating behavior.

Most of us with weight problems don't eat because of our appetites. We eat because of our anxieties.

Anxiety-induced eating doesn't actually relieve or dissolve the stress and anxiety that started the eating behavior.

Rather, anxiety-induced (over)eating serves merely as a temporary coping mechanism.

Because we're responding to how our emotions "eat" us, food becomes a kind of escape, as well as a temporary relaxant. Food and overeating become safety valves for our aroused emotions.

But for emotionally caused eating behavior, the chain of emotions doesn't stop with the last mouthful of food. The emotions that the eating has been used to suppress once again rise to the surface, this time in the form of guilt and shame for overeating. In this way, emotional overeating serves simultaneously as punishment and as reward. And this perpetuates a cycle of anxiety followed by eating followed by guilt (anxiety) followed by eating. It's a very tough cycle to break.

This syndrome, described above in a simplified form, is known by many names. Psychologists have called it bulimia (emotionally caused overeating); physiologists have called it stress-induced hyperphagia (overconsumption). In this book, we'll refer to this problem as compulsive/emotional eating.

Compulsive/emotional eating is one of the most prevalent and least diagnosed conditions in America. Compulsive/emotional eating afflicts most of the 80 million Americans who are more than ten pounds overweight. In a way, compulsive/emotional eating is similar to alcoholism or drug addiction. However, it would be incorrect to say that compulsive/emotional eaters are "addicted to food." Rather, they have an obsessive-compulsive relationship with food and eating. This doesn't mean they have a genuine physiological addiction to food in general or to specific "trigger" foods. Chocolate ice cream can't be considered addictive, even though you can't stop eating it. But chocolate ice cream could very well be a food that elicits strong emotional/compulsive reactions from you or other overeaters. And in this way, that chocolate ice cream is just as crucial to your condition as vodka is to an alcoholic or heroin is to a drug addict.

Let's make it clear, however, that possessing the compulsive/emotional eating syndrome *does not mean that you are mentally ill.* Rather, compulsive/emotional eating may be seen as a part of your overall personality structure. Just as some people are neat and other people are sloppy, some people are compulsives and others are not.

Having a compulsion-prone personality can manifest itself in other ways besides eating. Some compulsives express their personality structure in relatively innocuous ways. They may compulsively clean their houses, make lists, wash their hands, or pay their bills early. Or they may compulsively smoke, gamble—or overeat. You may have more compulsive behavior patterns besides overeating. But it's compulsive/emotional overeating that concerns you most, because its effects are most visible and the overweight often caused by compulsive/emotional eating is a stigma in this thin-obsessed society.

## WHAT IS A COMPULSION?

In a way, a compulsion is a habit. But compulsion is stronger than habit. You can get rid of a habit if you refrain from doing the habitual activity or if you *rationally* tell yourself over and over again that you must not do it. But a compulsion will remain as strong as ever, lurking in your subconscious, even if you refrain from doing it and logically prove to yourself that the compulsion is harmful to you and must be stopped.

What sets up and perpetuates a compulsion?

1. You encounter one or more emotional pains that must be deadened somehow. Or you may have situations that must be escaped. Or energy that must be worked off, dissipated, or concealed. Or thoughts and desires that must be forgotten or suppressed.

2. Given these emotional problems, the compulsion-prone person accidentally discovers an activity or group of activities that make him feel better. These activities may

temporarily mask his pain, dissipate the excess energy, or provide an escape.

These activities and groups of activities are the compulsive acts. Examples of compulsions include washing up, cleaning house, reorganizing files, making lists, working excessively (the workaholic syndrome), smoking, gambling, overeating, drinking.

3. After the emotionally deadening compulsive activities have been discovered by a compulsion-prone person, this person will continue to engage in compulsive activities whenever he feels emotional pain, excessive energy, or undesirable thoughts.

After a while, the compulsive-prone person begins to think, "If only I could eat/smoke/clean/overwork, *then* I'm sure I'd feel better."

The compulsion-prone person isn't exactly sure *why* he feels temporarily better after these compulsive activities, but he does know that they work—at least for a little while.

4. Gradually, the idea of doing this compulsive activity intrudes on the person's thoughts. When the compulsive activity comes to be thought of frequently or even dominates the person's thoughts, these compulsive activities become *obsessions*.

The obsessive thoughts demand that the compulsive activity must be performed, even if the compulsion-prone person knows that activity is silly, unnecessary, or even harmful.

Remember, all the time, the compulsive activity is not being performed for its own sake but to quiet some other emotional pain or problem.

5. After the compulsive activity has been performed, the relief is over. But now guilt, shame, more anxiety, and fears of not being in control take over. These emotions create more pain, more anxiety, and again stir up the need to deal with these emotional pains. This sets off the obsessive/compulsive cycle once again.

Eventually, the compulsion-prone person reaches the

point where he *must* perform the compulsive activity—*even though he doesn't want to do it.*

This is why so many compulsive/emotional eaters are unable to stop overeating, even though they know they shouldn't eat so much, even though they sincerely want to stop overeating. The obsessive/compulsive syndrome operates so strongly within these compulsive/emotional eaters that stopping their overeating is largely out of their conscious control.

When you behave in an obsessive/compulsive manner, you lose much of your freedom of choice. You then don't do things just because you consciously *want* to, but because you *have* to. Impelled by obsessive/compulsive patterns on a subconscious level, you feel you *must* perform your compulsive activity or "something terrible" will happen. That "something terrible" may be a feeling of escalating panic or an anxiety attack or a bout of depression. Or, worst of all, you may have to confront what's really bothering you—the emotional problems and pains that set off the compulsive response.

A longtime compulsive person may not be consciously aware of the emotional triggers that set his compulsive activities into motion. For a person with entrenched compulsions, the compulsive activity may start in *anticipation* of the problem and the pain. Thus, this person may short-circuit feelings of pain, but he also spends a lot of time doing compulsive acts he'd really rather not do, like smoking or overeating.

## COMPULSIONS ARE UNIMAGINATIVE

Compulsive behavior isn't the real problem. The compulsive behavior is a mask that the problem hides behind.

Religion may be "the opiate of the masses," but compulsive behavior is the opiate of the emotions in turmoil, in pain, rage, or fear. And, like an opiate or a narcotic, the compulsive behavior becomes *irresistible*, a kind of psychological addiction.

Why does this happen? Because the compulsion-prone individual feels he can't deal with life if he doesn't perform his compulsive activities. Too many tensions would well up and threaten to explode, threaten to destroy the precarious emotional equilibrium that the compulsion holds together.

Psychoanalysts have long held that compulsive behavior is merely the symptom of underlying problems. This theory of compulsive behavior is only partially true when it comes to food and (over)eating. That's because the psychoanalytic theory of compulsion doesn't take into account the extensive cultural, social, and media indoctrination which every member of this society has received regarding food and eating.

For many people, compulsive/emotional eating is the result of knowing only limited ways of dealing with emotional pain, grief, excess energy, or "bad" thoughts. So for the majority of people with weight problems, compulsive/emotional eating isn't so much psychoneurotic as it is *unimaginative*, a socially conditioned response to a given emotional situation.

A person with the compulsive/emotional eating syndrome is usually *limited in his repertoire of coping strategies*. He doesn't really know of any other ways of dealing with his problem or of enduring or lessening his emotional traumas.

Anyway, even if alternative modes of behavior are presented to an entrenched compulsive/emotional eater, none of those activities seems so "right," so effective, so satisfying, so irresistible, so inevitable as compulsive/emotional eating.

After all, we have grown used to compulsive/emotional eating since infancy. The syndrome began the very first time your mother gave you a bottle to quiet your infant cries. Compulsive/emotional eating dug in to stay when your parents gave you a lollipop when you fell and scraped your knee, and when they celebrated your birthday with a sticky-sweet cake and ice cream.

Compulsive/emotional eating occurs at every turn, every trauma, every joy in our lives from infancy onward. No wonder it's such an excruciatingly difficult cycle to break!

74

## COMPULSIVE/EMOTIONAL EATING AS ANESTHESIA

One of the most important functions of compulsive/emotional eating is to act as a general, all-purpose emotional anesthetic.

The compulsive/emotional eater "eats" the emotions of rage, anger, guilt, jealousy, and anxiety that he feels. Any strong emotion that the compulsive/emotional eater feels afraid to assert or to confront can be "eaten"—both symbolically and literally.

The very act of eating can be used to dull emotions, to deaden the emotions' intensity. How? By biting, chewing, licking, slicing, and sucking. In these actions, the compulsive/emotional eater can *safely* express some of his emotions, as well as dissipate some of the nervous tension and energy that are bottled up inside him.

## COMPONENTS OF COMPULSIVE/EMOTIONAL EATING

Each compulsive/emotional eater is a unique case. Each has a subtly different response, triggered by subtly different emotional, social, and cultural cues.

However, there are some elements that most compulsive/emotional eaters have in common:

1. Frequent preoccupation with thoughts of food and/or overweight.

2. Eating and overeating when not hungry—or even when feeling full or stuffed.

3. Erratic self-control around food. This lack of control can be either suppressed (this becomes dieting) or expressed (this becomes gorging or overeating).

4. Lack of self-esteem because of continually being on the verge of losing self-control regarding food, eating, and body size.

5. Often the above elements are accompanied by contempt for one's body or by simply feeling uncomfortable inside that body.

6. Often underestimation of the connection between eating and body size accompanies the other compulsive/emotional eating components. This means that the compulsive/emotional eater logically *knows* that overeating leads to overweight. But emotionally, he never quite makes the connection between what goes into the mouth and what bulges on the body.

## *DIETING AS A COMPULSION*

Dieting can become obsessive/compulsive behavior, too. The most obvious example of this occurs in people who are afflicted with the psychological disorder known as anorexia nervosa. These people literally can't *stop* dieting. They waste away, and even die, because they have an obsessive compulsion to diet stringently and to lose more and more weight.

But dieting can be obsessive/compulsive in much less severe forms. Compulsive dieting can manifest itself in the common quest for a miracle cure for overweight, for a "final solution" diet that will get the pounds off and keep them off permanently.

The obsessive/compulsive pattern of dieting is exemplified by the Duchess of Windsor's dictum "You can never be too rich or too thin." Since you can never be "too thin," theoretically you have to stay on a perpetual diet, in order to maintain fashionable slenderness. For such people—and they are legion—dieting becomes a way of life, a life-style that is every bit as much a result of obsessions and compulsions as is compulsive/emotional eating.

In this way, dieting and compulsive/emotional eating can be seen as two sides of the same coin. Both eating and not eating (dieting) can be compulsive. Both eating and not eating may be activities largely beyond the control of the obsessive/compulsive person, whose compulsions have robbed him of freedom of choice in these matters. An eating binge is the obvious compulsive act. But dieting is the less obvious compulsive act—an atonement for the first compulsion of overeating.

## LEVELS OF COMPULSIVE/EMOTIONAL EATING

Compulsive/emotional eating is not a black-and-white affair. There are many shades of gray, too.

Not everyone is equally compulsive about eating and overeating. The degree of severity of compulsive/emotional eating can vary drastically from one person to another. Some people are only mildly and occasionally compulsive/emotional in their eating, while other people have elevated anxiety-induced overeating into a whole life-style. You can test your own degree of compulsive/emotional eating in the self-scoring quiz in the next chapter.

However, degrees or levels of compulsive/emotional eating can be summarized here. The degree of compulsivity in an individual's eating can be judged by how often food and eating appear in the individual's life as an emotional response.

The level of a person's compulsive/emotional eating behavior can also be determined by:

1. The degree to which he accepts compulsive/emotional eating as irresistible, inevitable, or inescapable.

2. The severity of his binges (how much is consumed, how long the binge lasts).

3. The frequency of the binges and uncontrollable, compulsive/emotional eating. (How often does bingeing or chaotic eating occur? Every day, every week, every month?) How much of the individual's time is spent trying to overcome or atone for compulsive/emotional eating?

4. The degree to which compulsive/emotional eating has become a part of the individual's life-style.

5. The degree to which compulsive/emotional eating imparts meaning to the individual's life (how much he lives to eat, instead of eats to live).

## WHO ARE THE COMPULSIVE EATERS?

Here we're going to introduce you to four compulsive/emotional eaters. For some, compulsive/emotional eating is a minor part of their lives. For others, compulsive/emotional eating is a dominating force in their and their families' lives.

These personality sketches show a progression in compulsive/emotional eating, a growth of severity in the condition. We begin with Louise, who uses compulsive/emotional eating in response to specific anxieties, and we end with Paul, who displays compulsive/emotional eating at its most severe, at which point compulsive/emotional eating becomes an all-encompassing life-style; compulsive/emotional eating runs Paul's life and eliminates most of his freedom of choice *not* to eat.

### Louise, a mild compulsive/emotional eater

To look at Louise, you would never guess that she has an eating problem. She is a slender 122 pounds and 5 feet 9 inches tall. Louise looks like a model; in fact, she is one, specializing in television commercials and photographic ads. Yet this willowy woman is frequently obsessed by food. She binges on sweets and junk foods, in particular.

"When I'm under a lot of stress, I'll gobble down anything in sight," Louise admits. "To avoid overeating, I've found that I can't keep anything in my refrigerator at home at all. I have to eat all my meals out in restaurants. That way, there's nothing at home for me to gorge myself on."

This ingenious system works only part of the time, however. Because during two or three tension-wrought days each month, Louise sneaks down to the A & P and buys a dozen chocolate-covered doughnuts and a quart of maple syrup. "I hate to admit it, but I eat it all at one sitting," she says, shaking her head. "I find that I eat all these ultra-sweet things until I feel sleepy. Then I fall into bed and sleep it off, as if I were a drunk sleeping off his liquor."

Louise uses compulsive/emotional eating two or three days each month to achieve emotional anesthesia—she literally sedates herself with her brief but massive carbohydrate intake.

"I went to my doctor and told him about my cravings for maple syrup, but he just laughed at me," Louise reports. "He said it wasn't so unusual. He had a few women patients who did the same thing just before or during their menstrual periods. He told me not to worry, because I wasn't gaining weight, just eating myself sick occasionally.

"If he only knew *how* I keep those binges from putting weight on me!" Louise sighs. "The day after I've binged, I get so disgusted with myself, I don't eat at all. Just black coffee and grapefruit until I've knocked off the couple of pounds that one miserable binge has put on me."

Louise can't make the connection in her mind between her occasional eating binges and her emotions. She honestly can't figure out afterward why it was that she ate like such a pig, completely out of control for hours at a time. Louise would be shocked to hear that she, a professional skinny, a model, is a mild compulsive/emotional eater.

### Andrea, a moderate or average compulsive/emotional eater

A fifth-grade teacher with two school-age children of her own, Andrea lives on a continual binge-to-famine eating cycle. She feels she's always poised on the brink of giving in to her irrational desire to eat and eat and eat. Because of her binges, Andrea is always "atoning" for her eating transgressions. Her weight seesaws up and down—ten pounds up, ten pounds down.

"I don't know why I lack willpower," Andrea moans. "I try, I really try, to keep my eating under control. But sometimes, I just go berserk and take the kids to McDonald's and eat a caramel sundae and a bag of fries along with them. And that, right after I've *vowed* to stick to my diet for another week. I just hate it when I overeat that way, so I go right back on my diet the next day. That's how it is with me: off again, on again, always either on a diet, breaking a diet, or getting psyched up to go on another diet. It's a hell of a way to live."

Andrea is devoted to women's magazines and regularly tries out the latest diet she finds in their pages. Over the years, she has been on the Atkins Diet Revolution, Weight Watchers, the Stillman water diet, the Mayo Clinic diet, Diet Watchers program, and, currently, the fructose no-hunger diet. With all her dieting, you'd think Andrea had a serious weight problem. She doesn't. She weighs about 135 pounds most of the time, but longs to have only 118 pounds on her 5-foot-5-inch frame.

"No matter how much I diet, no matter how long I diet, I can never quite make it down to my goal weight," Andrea sighs. "I'm always on the lookout for some new diet break-through that will help me crack that five-pounds-above-goal barrier. Someday, I swear, I'll make it."

Besides her private attempts at dieting, Andrea once consulted an endocrinologist, to see if hormonal modifications could keep her weight down. "He told me I *might* be able to get thinner, if he removed my ovaries. I said, 'Thanks but no thanks.' I would do almost anything to get thin, but that's going a bit too far, even for me."

Some of the modifications Andrea has made in her lifestyle to compensate for her binge days of overeating include always drinking skim milk; using only saccharin as a sweetener; eating all her sandwiches open-face; using only diet dressing on her salads.

Still, Andrea does wax rapturous when she tells of her favorite binge foods: "Pizza! I could eat pizza all day long—anchovy pizza, pepperoni pizza, mushroom pizza. It's my favorite thing in the world." Embarrassed, she admits that she always drinks diet soda with her binge pizzas: "I've got to cut down on calories somewhere."

Andrea is concerned about "fat-proofing" her kids. "I don't want them to have my overeating problems," she says. "But despite everything I've tried to teach them, they both love junk food and sweets a lot more than they love proteins and vegetables."

Whether she realizes it or not, Andrea is a typical dieter. She exemplifies the moderate or average degree of compulsive/emotional eating. Andrea doesn't realize that she might be a somewhat compulsive eater; all she knows is that she has shaky willpower. She's convinced that if she can "tough it out," she'll eventually—someday, somehow—diet herself down to gloriously bony thinness. "All I need is a little more willpower and a better diet," she concludes.

### Fran, an entrenched compulsive/emotional eater

You can immediately *see* that Fran has both a weight problem and an overeating problem. An attractive woman in her fifties, Fran stands 5 feet 3 inches tall but weighs 155 pounds. She was always a few pounds overweight, but in the past ten years, since her youngest child went off to college, Fran has gained about twenty pounds. She can't seem to get the excess weight off.

Diets used to work for her, "but now I just don't have the willpower or the guts to stick it out on a diet. I just tend to let myself slide. I sit at home all day, so naturally I end up eating too much. I guess I'm bored, although sometimes I feel as if my nerves were going to snap from sheer tension."

Like Andrea, Fran is a veteran of the Diet Wars. For years, she kept a vigilant eye on her weight as registered on the bathroom scale. She has lost weight at TOPS and at health clubs. She has starved on the liquid-protein diet and on a "sensible" thousand-calorie-a-day regimen her family doctor prescribed. Fran has also gone to diet doctors twice. Each time, she was given a bottleful of amphetamines and diuretic pills and a stringent diet of 600 to 800 calories.

One of the diet doctors also gave her shots of hormones from pregnant cows. "It was supposed to speed up the weight loss," Fran recalls, "and, for a while, it seemed to work. I looked just beautiful after I finished that doctor's program. But a year and a half later, I had gained all the weight back. I was so embarrassed, I didn't have enough nerve to go back to that doctor, so I tried to put myself on a diet. That worked pretty well, too. But I gained the weight back again."

Fran grimaces. "It's been like that my whole life, ever since I was a young girl. Always on a diet. I'd lose the weight, then gain it back. So I'd try another diet, lose the weight, and gain it back again. About five years ago, I got fed up with dieting. I figured that I would just try to enjoy food for once in my life, instead of feeling guilty every time I ate a morsel. So I proceeded to enjoy my food for six months, and I overate so badly, I ended up like a sausage stuffed into my clothes. I tried to get back on one of my strict diets, but I just couldn't bring myself to go through all that deprivation and worrying about calories again."

At present, Fran puts herself on a diet two or three times a year, but she quits after a few weeks and a five- or six-pound weight loss. Her eating style might be described as chaotic—binges some days and apathy toward food on other days.

Compulsive/emotional eating has become an integral part of Fran's life-style, even though she would be surprised to hear herself described as an entrenched compulsive/emotional eater. She spends more time, on average, involved in compulsive/emotional eating than not involved in it. By now, she eats in anticipation of emotional stress, without even realizing what she's doing.

**Paul, an extreme compulsive/emotional eater**

For years, Paul has referred to himself jovially as "a man who throws a lot of weight around in Massachusetts politics, both literally and figuratively." A lawyer by profession, Paul is the mayor of a small city, a devoted husband, and the father of four. At 6 feet tall, he weighs 325 pounds. Paul is an extremely severe case of compulsive/emotional eating, but no one has ever diagnosed this as being his problem. He views himself as an undisciplined slob, even though he worked his way through law school and was respected enough to be elected to several state and city offices, despite his girth.

"My mama didn't go, 'Eat, eat,' like most Italian mothers," Paul recalls. "She· would take all the fat off my meats and cook the meat in plain water to cut down calories. She'd put one small spoonful of macaroni with sauce on my plate. She told me to eat greens, things that would satisfy the mouth but not add more pounds. But I still stayed fat.

"I would eat one of my mother's well-balanced meals and then go straight to the corner diner and eat five sandwiches, Cokes, coleslaw, fries. I became a balloon. It wasn't Italian food that killed me. It was American delicatessen and Cokes and fries that did it to me."

Paul's massive overeating is reminiscent of an anecdote told by the portly film director Orson Welles: "My doctor has advised me to give up those intimate little dinners for four—unless there are three other people eating with me."

Despite being fifty pounds overweight, Paul found a woman to love and marry him. He ate huge amounts while he stayed up nights, studying for law school and later for his bar exams. "I figure the bar exams alone added twenty-five pounds onto me. I was eating for strength, for success, and because I was scared to death."

Years later, as mayor of his small Massachusetts city, Paul still found himself using food as a reward and as consolation. He dieted sporadically, but soon grew discouraged and gave up: "I could lose twenty-five, thirty pounds, and I'd still look fat. It seemed hopeless."

So Paul found himself eating like this: "After a day in which I thought I was a particularly good mayor—I had solved a lot of problems, done a lot of people favors—I'd go to the grocery before I went home and load up on a whole prosciutto, a whole mozzarella, a couple of loaves of bread, some other goodies. Then I'd go home and go straight up to my study and lock the door. I laid the food out in a row in front of me on my desk, and while I read law books or watched TV, I'd finish everything I had brought home. Then I would go downstairs and eat a full meal with my family.

"It's terrible to admit, but I used to lock the door so my kids couldn't get in and take part of my reward food. I love my kids, and yet I couldn't make myself share that food with them. It made me feel rotten, like a despicable person."

Eventually, however, it was love for his children that gave Paul the emotional fortitude to attempt a very strict, doctor-prescribed liquid diet: "I thought, What if I die from overweight? How will my children remember me? As a fat man who died, because he drowned in his own fat? That was an incentive for me to diet. My doctor figured out that I was eating ten thousand calories a day at my peak weight!"

Paul's history showed the classic components of compulsive/emotional eating. He followed a predictable cycle of binge, starve, binge, starve, and also a cycle of punish (deprive by diet), reward, punish, reward. All these feelings were acted out in his relationships to food and eating.

Paul displays another classic set of attitudes of the compulsive/emotional overeater: he is filled with self-hate, self-contempt, and self-reproach.

You can read between the lines to see these emotions in another of Paul's statements: "If you see a fat person, you see a weak person. I feel fat means you're not mature. It means you're deserving of contempt for your weakness. When I look in the mirror, I see my whole bloated body. I see how disgustingly fat and ugly I am. Other people see it and despise me, too. When people get mad at me, the first thing they'll call me is a fat slob."

Paul's life has not been an easy one. Although he showed the competence and dedication to succeed as a lawyer and politician, Paul can see only his failings—his overweight. This promotes such severe feelings of worthlessness and self-hate that these negative feelings set off yet another cycle of severe compulsive/emotional eating. Then Paul berates himself for his supposed lack of willpower, for his supposed weakness and immaturity. Actually, Paul's achievements show that he has tremendous self-discipline, inner strength, and maturity.

But how can Paul succeed at permanently losing weight when he hates himself?

# RECENT FINDINGS ON THE PSYCHOLOGY
# OF OVEREATING

Scientific research on overeating and obesity has recently begun to challenge old theories on overweight. No longer do social scientists think that the overweight person is a psychological weakling. Rather, the overweight-prone person has been shown to be a person whose emotions are powerful and long-lasting.

Studies conducted by Drs. Donald Elman and Stanley Schachter of Columbia University and Dr. Judith Rodin of Yale University have found that overweight people generally eat more when they are emotionally aroused by either positive or negative emotions. That means that almost any emotion—joy, rage, boredom, fear—can trigger eating in a person prone to overweight. The Elman-Schachter-Rodin studies also showed that obese people's emotions are more easily aroused than those of normal-weight people.

Other research by Dr. Jules Hirsch of New York's Rockefeller University gives clues as to why overweight people find it so emotionally difficult—or impossible—to stay on diets. Hirsch found that when obese people lose large amounts of weight, many of them become "depressed and anxious." Many such people, Hirsch says, feel "deprived, left out, lonesome, and empty in a global sense." In other words, Hirsch found that when on a long-term diet and losing many pounds, obese people react in a way that is similar to that of normal-weight people who are starving. It's difficult to keep on a diet when you're receiving the severe emotional/physical messages of starvation!

Even the stern, constant vigilance that many dieters exercise may contribute to their failure at weight loss. Rodin of Yale believes that dieters' "continual restraint" leads them to feel *compelled* by food until their self-control weakens. Rodin concluded that overweight people, in order to keep their weight down, should "get off diets as such and learn to live more normally with food."

Another psychologist, Dr. Richard Nisbett, has done research that leads him to believe that obesity is biologically determined. All people have an inner body programming to remain at a certain weight, a weight that Nisbett terms their "biological set point." Overweight people on diets are chronically below their biological set point. Thus, according to Nisbett's theory, these dieters are always literally starving, even though they may be above the actuarial tables' "ideal" weights. Overweight people on diets are literally starving, so it's no wonder that they pay so much attention to food. According to Nisbett's reasoning, a naturally obese person who attempts to reduce is dooming himself to failure by the simple act of dieting, an act that his body interprets as real starvation, not just temporary food deprivation.

Research recently announced by two scientists from the Mount Sinai School of Medicine, City University of New York—Drs. Eugene Straus and Nobel Prize winner Rosalyn S. Yalow—indicates that brain chemistry may be the original cause for much of what we call compulsive/emotional eating. Straus and Yalow believe that the nerve-regulating brain chemical cholecystokinin may be linked to overweight.

For many years, it's been known that damage to the hypothalamus (a brain center where cholecystokinin occurs) is typically associated with obesity. Straus and Yalow have found that genetically obese, overeating mice have only 25 to 33 percent as much cholecystokinin in their brains as do nonobese, nonovereating mice. Straus and Yalow hypothesize that these low levels of cholecystokinin in the obese, overeating mice's brains may be the direct cause of their "unrestrained appetites."

It's a bit of a leap from fat mice to compulsive/emotional-overeating human beings. But the ultimate implication of the Straus-Yalow research may be that a low level of brain chemicals could be the *real* reason you just can't stop eating and eating and eating.

It will be many years, if ever, before the findings of Straus, Yalow, Nisbett, Rodin, Elman, Schachter, and other researchers can be applied to help human beings with over-eating and overweight problems. Until then, we can only attempt to work with the simple tools we already have for dealing with overeating and overweight—tools like diet, exercise, and changes in life-style and mental attitude.

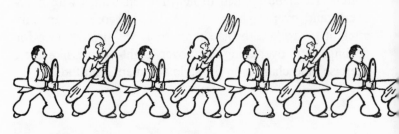

# 6 Are You a Compulsive/ Emotional Eater?

Did you recognize yourself in the brief character sketches of compulsive/emotional eaters that appeared in the last chapter? Do you feel you eat because of anxiety, instead of appetite? Is overeating a part of your life-style, not just an occasional binge?

One good way to judge accurately how much of a compulsive/emotional eater you are is to take the self-scoring test that begins below. This quiz is designed to help you gauge your own, personal degree of compulsive/emotional eating. It should also help you to uncover and identify some of the emotional triggers that cause you to overeat.

As you take this self-test, mark your answers directly on the pages of the book. That way, you'll be able to go back over the quiz at your leisure and analyze your answers, figure out just what causes your (over)eating behavior.

After the quiz questions, there's a section telling how to score the test yourself—and how to interpret those scores. You'll be able to determine just how much compulsive and emotional dimensions in your personality contribute to your eating and overeating. But remember—the important thing about this test isn't how many points you score but how honest you can be with yourself. The goal of taking this self-scoring quiz isn't to shame you or to make you hate yourself so you'll change your ways; the goal is to know yourself better. This increased self-knowledge may give you an improved ability to diagnose and solve your own eating problems.

Circle your answer to each question below.

## EMOTIONAL EATING TRIGGERS

1. Do you feel compelled to eat something after you've had an argument with someone who means a lot to you?

   Never    Seldom    Sometimes    Often    Almost always

2. Do you *need* to eat when you feel worried or depressed or tense?

   Never    Seldom    Sometimes    Often    Almost always

3. Is your idea of a "reward" a special food, or going out to eat, or splurging on a calorie-rich dessert or starchy ethnic food?

   Never    Seldom    Sometimes    Often    Almost always

4. When you think about a food or get a food yen, can you delay eating or avoid eating altogether?

   Never    Seldom    Sometimes    Often    Almost always

5. How often do you give yourself a reward (a present to yourself) of something other than food?

   Never    Seldom    Sometimes    Often    Almost always

6. You're on a diet. Your hostess or a friend you're lunching with insists that you eat some forbidden, high-calorie food like a sundae or a slice of pie. How often do you give in to this kind of pressure—perhaps even with a secret feeling of relief, because you now have an excuse to break or bend your diet?

   Never    Seldom    Sometimes    Often    Almost always

7. You've sampled a high-calorie food or a food forbidden on your diet. Does that "sample taste" set you off on a major or minor eating binge?

    Never    Seldom    Sometimes    Often    Almost always

8. You walk by a bakery or a candy shop. Can you resist going into that shop and buying a pastry or sweets?

    Never    Seldom    Sometimes    Often    Almost always

9. You have steered clear of that bakery or candy shop or some other source of temptation. Soon afterward, do you feel edgy and end up yielding to temptation by eating something "forbidden"?

    Never    Seldom    Sometimes    Often    Almost always

10. Do you eat foods that you *know* are "bad" for you?

    Never    Seldom    Sometimes    Often    Almost always

11. Did your parents reward you with sweets?

    Never    Seldom    Sometimes    Often    Almost always

12. How frequently do you feel that if you eat something, you'll feel better?

    Never    Seldom    Sometimes    Often    Almost always

13. You feel angry or frustrated or hostile. Does this make you want to eat or overeat?

    Never    Seldom    Sometimes    Often    Almost always

14. You feel worn out. Do you eat to invigorate yourself?

    Never    Seldom    Sometimes    Often    Almost always

## EATING PATTERNS

15. Do you gulp down your food, instead of chewing slowly and/or savoring its taste?

    Never    Seldom    Sometimes    Often    Almost always

16. Do you feel you *have* to eat at certain times of the day besides mealtimes? For instance, just before bedtime, at coffee breaks, before the kids come home from school?

Never     Seldom     Sometimes     Often     Almost always

17. Do you ever feel surprised that you've eaten so much without really noticing what went into your mouth—just shovel it in without really thinking?

Never     Seldom     Sometimes     Often     Almost always

18. Do you prefer to eat alone because food tastes better that way, because then you can let your inhibitions down about how much and what kind of food you eat?

Never     Seldom     Sometimes     Often     Almost always

19. How often do you put yourself on a diet to lose weight and then find yourself breaking the diet rather quickly, uncontrollably?

Never     Seldom     Sometimes     Often     Almost always

20. Do you have eating binges that last for several days at a time?

Never     Seldom     Sometimes     Often     Almost always

21. Do you plan ahead of time to have secret/solo eating binges?

Never     Seldom     Sometimes     Often     Almost always

22. How often do you find yourself eating even though you're not really hungry?

Never     Seldom     Sometimes     Often     Almost always

23. Do you eat sensibly when you're dining in the company of others but gorge/binge afterward when you're alone?

Never     Seldom     Sometimes     Often     Almost always

24. How often do you go on an eating binge?

Never     Seldom     Sometimes     Often     Almost always

**25.** Do you stuff yourself or gorge until you feel uncomfortably full?

Never     Seldom     Sometimes     Often     Almost always

**26.** Do you get uncontrollable desires for foods or uncontrollable urges to eat?

Never     Seldom     Sometimes     Often     Almost always

**27.** Have you ever woken up in the middle of the night and had a strong *need* to eat before you can fall back to sleep?

Never     Seldom     Sometimes     Often     Almost always

**28.** Do you feel you must eat in secret?

Never     Seldom     Sometimes     Often     Almost always

**29.** Do you hide foods, so that you can keep them for yourself alone?

Never     Seldom     Sometimes     Often     Almost always

**30.** You feel really full. Do you eat anyway?

Never     Seldom     Sometimes     Often     Almost always

**31.** Do you stockpile food, especially your favorite binge foods—just to make sure you don't run out?

Never     Seldom     Sometimes     Often     Almost always

**32.** Do you find that you haven't actually tasted the food that you've eaten?

Never     Seldom     Sometimes     Often     Almost always

**33.** How frequently do you eat standing up?

Never     Seldom     Sometimes     Often     Almost always

**34.** Do you find that there are some foods that you just can't stop eating?

Never     Seldom     Sometimes     Often     Almost always

## FEELINGS ABOUT EATING HABITS

35. Do you feel guilty about your eating habits and eating patterns?

Never    Seldom    Sometimes    Often    Almost always

36. How often do you try to kid yourself by saying, "I really don't eat that much"?

Never    Seldom    Sometimes    Often    Almost always

37. Are you annoyed when your friends or family tell you that you're overeating or that you "really need to take off a few pounds"?

Never    Seldom    Sometimes    Often    Almost always

38. Are you embarrassed to let other people see you eating in public places, such as restaurants, school or company cafeterias, parties?

Never    Seldom    Sometimes    Often    Almost always

39. Some people eat to live. Others live to eat. How often do you find yourself "living for the sake of eating"?

Never    Seldom    Sometimes    Often    Almost always

40. Do you feel you're struggling to keep your appetite under control?

Never    Seldom    Sometimes    Often    Almost always

41. You can't concentrate on an important assignment. You have a snack, because you'll be able to think better after you've had something to eat. How often have you done this?

Never    Seldom    Sometimes    Often    Almost always

42. You're eating out with other people at a restaurant. Do you feel you should just pick at your food, because a person like you shouldn't eat too much—especially in public?

Never    Seldom    Sometimes    Often    Almost always

43. Are there periods of time when eating is one of the major joys in your life?

Never    Seldom    Sometimes    Often    Almost always

44. You're hungry and pick up something to eat. Your spouse/parent/friend tells you, "Don't eat so much. Stick to your diet." You stop eating in his presence. But later you make a point of eating something when he can't see you, just to prove that you're not going to let other people run your life. How often have you done this?

Never    Seldom    Sometimes    Often    Almost always

45. How often do you think about your weight problem or about your eating patterns of diet, binge, diet, binge?

Never    Seldom    Sometimes    Often    Almost always

46. Do your weight problems or your food compulsions make you or your loved ones unhappy?

Never    Seldom    Sometimes    Often    Almost always

47. How often do you think about your degree of over-weight or overeating?

Never    Seldom    Sometimes    Often    Almost always

48. Do you scan the latest fad and wonder diets, looking for some kind of miracle solution to your weight and eating problems?

Never    Seldom    Sometimes    Often    Almost always

49. There are no sweets or ice cream or other binge foods in your house today. You fear that you might go up the wall or actually crack up tonight, because you have nothing to nibble on. How often has this happened to you?

Never    Seldom    Sometimes    Often    Almost always

50. Which of these alternatives would you *honestly* prefer?
    a. a good night's sleep

b. making love, culminating in an orgasm
c. a good meal with a friend or lover
d. a solitary binge with all your favorite foods

## SELF-ESTEEM

51. Are you ashamed of the way your body looks?

Never     Seldom     Sometimes     Often     Almost always

52. Have you avoided having a medical examination because you're afraid the doctor will tell you to go on a diet?

Never     Seldom     Sometimes     Often     Almost always

53. Have you avoided seeing old friends because you were ashamed of how much weight you've put on?

Never     Seldom     Sometimes     Often     Almost always

54. Have you ever postponed buying new clothes because you're ashamed of your shape/size/weight and hate the way clothes look on you?

Never     Seldom     Sometimes     Often     Almost always

55. Do your overeating habits make you feel that you're lacking in self-control and, hence, are an inferior person?

Never     Seldom     Sometimes     Often     Almost always

56. Do you ever mistreat yourself or want to punish yourself?

Never     Seldom     Sometimes     Often     Almost always

57. Are you afraid you'll gain weight?

Never     Seldom     Sometimes     Often     Almost always

58. "If I could just get rid of this overeating problem, I'd look better and feel better, and my whole life would be so much happier." How often do you feel as if this statement applies to you?

Never     Seldom     Sometimes     Often     Almost always

**59.** Are you kinder or nicer to other people than you are to yourself?

Never    Seldom    Sometimes    Often    Almost always

## SCORING

You can score a maximum of 295 points on this quiz. Use a separate sheet of paper or write in the margins of this book, whichever is more convenient for you in adding up your points.

For questions 4, 5, 7, and 8 *only*:

| | |
|---|---|
| Never | = 5 |
| Seldom | = 4 |
| Sometimes | = 3 |
| Often | = 2 |
| Almost always | = 1 |

For question 50 *only*:

| | |
|---|---|
| a | = 1 |
| b | = 1 |
| c | = 4 |
| d | = 5 |

For all other questions:

| | |
|---|---|
| Never | = 1 |
| Seldom | = 2 |
| Sometimes | = 3 |
| Often | = 4 |
| Almost always | = 5 |

## WHAT DOES YOUR SCORE MEAN?

**If you scored 102 points or less . . .**

You are the type of person who makes little or no connection between eating and your emotional state. You are not at all compulsive regarding your eating habits. For you, food is seen as fuel for the body, nothing more or less. Your eating habits probably fluctuate very little in response to your moods.

**If you scored 103–147 points . . .**

Emotions play a role in your eating and overeating, but that role is a relatively small one. You are only mildly affected by your emotions when you decide what, how much, and when to eat. For the most part, eating is a consciously controlled activity for you. Any emotional factors can be suppressed with comparative ease, so that your eating habits are more logical than the average person's.

**If you scored 148–177 points . . .**

You are in the average/normal range for emotional and compulsive components of your eating behavior. Your emotions do have an effect on how much you eat. Usually, your response to a negative emotion is to overeat somewhat. But if you are really depressed or under severe anxiety and stress, your emotions may actually put a damper on your eating, and then you may undereat.

Because emotions color your attitudes toward food, you probably have a more sensual nature regarding food, and under emotionally calm circumstances, eating can be a real source of sensory pleasure to you.

**If you scored 177–221 points . . .**

Your emotional/compulsive component regarding eating is somewhat higher than average. Any strong emotion can trigger a compulsive response that makes you want to eat. Because of this rather volatile emotional nature, you tend to put on weight easily. You go on and off diets several times each year. When you go off your diet, you berate yourself for a shortage of willpower.

However, what you consider your lack of willpower is actually the result of the strength of your emotions and compulsions regarding food and eating. At the same time, you do derive pleasure from foods' tastes, smells, and appearances. You are sensually attuned to food and enjoy a good meal in companionable surroundings.

**If you scored 222–250 points . . .**

You are an entrenched compulsive eater. Probably more than half your eating time is spent eating compulsively, for emotional reasons that you may not even be aware of. You use food, either consciously or unconsciously, as a kind of emotional anesthesia; food and overeating are primary means by which you "cope" with life's troubles.

When you are not on a diet, you are thinking about going on a diet. You feel you overeat too often, so you are filled with guilt and shame about your eating habits and your size and shape.

You may be comparatively slim, or you may be noticeably overweight. Either way, much of your time is spent thinking about food or about dieting. You often feel your eating is out of control. You can enjoy foods, but sometimes you eat so fast that you can't even taste what you're putting in your mouth.

**If you scored 250–295 points . . .**

You are an extremely compulsive eater. Emotional and compulsive drives set your mouth in action. Stress and anxiety steer you directly toward food. Eating is one of your primary responses to current or potential problems. You may use food to reward and punish yourself simultaneously.

Usually, with this degree of compulsivity in your eating, you have a noticeable weight problem. This, unfortunately, makes you feel even worse about yourself. Your self-esteem is very low, and this kind of emotional pain only serves to send you on another bout of compulsive eating. Overeating has become a kind of life-style for you. Your eating habits are chaotic and often out of your conscious control.

You may be an especially sensitive and vulnerable person, emotionally high-strung. Eating and overeating are your ways of protecting your fragile emotional state. You need compassion and help from your family and friends.

However, because of your low self-esteem and weight problem, you may feel you deserve no such help. In fact, you may feel you're an inferior person, and thus you become self-destructive. Then, eating may become your slow means of physical and emotional suicide.

Be kinder to yourself; don't berate yourself further if you got this score.

## NOW WHAT?

Through this self-scoring quiz, you have some idea now of how much emotions and compulsions affect your eating and overeating. You may be pleasantly surprised, if you're not as much of a compulsive eater as you thought. Or perhaps your quiz score confirms your suspicions that you *are* a compulsive eater to some degree. Or perhaps you're amazed that compulsive/emotional eating is a prominent factor in your eating and dieting.

Whatever your reaction to your test score, the next step is to pinpoint *how* you engage in your compulsive/emotional eating. All compulsive/emotional eaters don't (over)eat in the same ways. The following three chapters will show you a variety of overeating and undereating personality types. Keep on reading—and you'll probably recognize yourself in one or in several of those types. You'll find that those special or peculiar ways you eat and overeat aren't so special or so peculiar after all.

When it comes to compulsive/emotional eating, you are not alone. You're not one *in* a million; you're one *of* millions.

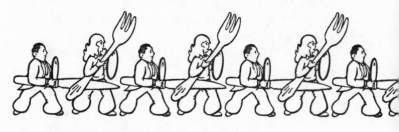

# 7 Eating Personalities: Overeaters, I

Since food "talks" to us so loudly, and since culture "talks" food so incessantly, it's no wonder that most of us overeat, even though we're dedicated to the lifelong Pursuit of Thin. It's the rare individual who doesn't succumb to overeating behavior patterns at one time or another. We give in to the urge to eat—and overeat—with so much guilt and shame that most people never realize that their own secret over-eating pattern really isn't so unusual after all. In fact, inter-viewing dozens of people—fat, thin, and in between—leads to the inescapable conclusion that overeating isn't just a momentary aberration; it's an integral part of most people's life-styles.

Once you realize that you're not alone in your "secret" overeating patterns, you can overcome some of the guilt and shame you feel after you've shoved a few thousand extra, unneeded calories down your throat. You can start to realize that all this guilt-laden overeating behavior is actually pretty funny. It's bizarre how most of us will go to such great lengths to conceal our overeating. We think we can keep that overeating a secret most of the time—even though the results of it are riding lumpily on hips, thighs, and abdomens. But it's even more ridiculous to believe that you're alone in your overeating pattern, no matter how seemingly strange that pattern may be. No matter *how* you overeat, you are not alone. You have thousands, perhaps millions, of fellow overeaters who share your supposedly idiosyncratic overeating patterns.

Some of the most common overeating personality types and patterns are described in this chapter and the next. As you glance through the two chapters analyzing and describing overeaters, you're probably going to recognize the personality types of your family members, your friends, your co-workers. And you'll probably find yourself and your own private eating aberrations, too. These case histories have been gleaned from dozens of interviews with people just like yourself.

What it all goes to prove is that nobody's perfect. Nobody *always* has good eating habits. No one *always* consumes a well-balanced, sensible diet. No one *always* possesses even minimal willpower. In eating (and overeating), willpower generally is overruled by wantpower. If you want to eat, you usually do. And sometimes you overeat even when you don't want to—for emotional reasons that operate largely on subconscious levels.

## HOW TO MAKE YOUR OWN PERSONAL EATING PERSONALITY PROFILE

Since no one is exclusively one type or another, it helps to construct your own Eating Personality Profile. This can be done easily by using a ten-point scale. As you read through the following eating-personality types, estimate the degree to which that personality type or eating syndrome is like yourself.

If you're not at all like that, mark a zero next to the personality type.

If you're like that very rarely, mark it 1.

Rarely = 2.

Very occasionally = 3.

Occasionally = 4.

Sometimes = 5.

Often = 6.
Frequently = 7.
Very frequently = 8.
Almost all the time = 9.
All the time = 10.

Write your evaluations of yourself—the numbers based on the ten-point scale—right in the box next to each eating-personality type. *Use* this book—don't just read it. Maintain your personal record on these pages.

Mark down your ten-point scale judgments based on how you're behaving with regard to food right now, at this point in your life. Don't make these judgments based on the way you used to behave, or on the way you'd like to behave. Be realistic. Tell yourself the truth. You may find you've got a little bit of the Rebel with a Cause in you, a lot of the Secret Snacker, and a soupçon of the Junk Food Junkie.

Once you make these judgments about your eating personality, you'll have an idea of the specific components of your eating behavior—and of your eating problem. Then you can make better, more accurate decisions on how to combat these tendencies within yourself. Or you can decide whether you'd be happier just learning to live with them.

People take their eating habits very seriously. They feel distressed when their eating habits are less than perfect. By understanding the diversity of eating personalities, you'll be able to see how laughable most people's eating patterns are. For these often nutty ways of living with food and eating aren't uncommon—they're typical.

Once you can see that your immense problems with food and eating are shared by thousands and thousands of other people, you can laugh at the strange ways you all torture yourselves with your good eating habits—or lack of them. And when you can laugh at yourself, you can stop being hung up about overeating or undereating, of staying on a diet or breaking a diet. You can laugh at all those worries and get on to more important things—like living a happier, more productive life, as we'll discuss in the last three chapters of this book.

# OVEREATING PERSONALITY TYPES

## The Rebel with a Cause ☐

This type of overeater has made a conspicuous attempt at losing weight. Sometimes this personality pattern surfaces when the diet is in full swing. Sometimes it erupts when the diet is long past and all the lost weight has been regained. The husband/wife/roommate/parents/friends/co-workers of the Rebel with a Cause tell him not to overeat. All of the Rebel's loved ones are after him to stop eating so much, to shed all that ugly avoirdupois and expose some bones again.

These spouses, friends, and family members are determined to do good, so they will personally monitor the Rebel's eating habits, tell him when he's eating too much, remind him rather caustically, "It was eating like that before that gave you a pot belly."

Instead of responding gratefully to all these admonitions to diet or at least to eat sensibly, the Rebel with a Cause reacts in just the opposite manner. The Rebel wants to show that he is in control of his own life, his own eating habits. He wants to show everyone who's bossing him around that *he's* in control of his food consumption, and that he cannot be controlled, dominated, or smothered by these well-meaning would-be authority figures.

So what does he do to show that he's in control of his overeating? The Rebel with a Cause goes on an eating binge.

Roy is a perfect example of the Rebel with a Cause. He was always ten or fifteen pounds overweight, even as a boy. His parents would nag Roy to eat properly, so that he could lose weight: "Drink skim milk. Don't eat those greasy french fries when you go out. No, you may not have a second helping—you've eaten quite enough, young man."

His parents' attempts to take control of his eating habits drove Roy straight up the wall. In typical adolescent fashion, he did exactly the opposite of what he was told to do. If his father told him to lay off the french fries, Roy would sneak down to the hamburger stand at the first opportunity and order fries. If his mother told him no second helpings at dinner until he lost some weight, Roy would buy two desserts the next day at the school cafeteria.

"I used to get so *mad!*" he recalls. "I was damned if anybody would tell me how to live my own life. Supposedly, we have the right to life, liberty, and the pursuit of happiness. Well, for me sometimes, the pursuit of happiness is the pursuit of food. And to deny me the amount and kind of food I want when I want it makes me want to revolt."

You would think Roy would grow out of this behavior as he left adolescence. He did for a while, but the Rebel with a Cause personality pattern had only been submerged. It resurfaced after Roy got married. His wife was well-meaning and decided to help Roy cut out high-cholesterol items from his daily diet to prevent heart disease. "The more my wife told me I shouldn't eat eggs and butter and red meat, the more I craved these foods, and the more I ate them. I think my cholesterol count got higher, not lower, because I would sometimes make a special point of ordering high-cholesterol foods when I ate out."

When his doctor—a powerful authority figure in Roy's eyes—ordered him to lose some weight as he entered his forties, Roy really rebelled. "I went on an eating binge that lasted for weeks. I just boiled when I saw the smug way that doctor was telling *me* not to eat and all the while he was patting his own paunch. Who did he think he was, telling me how to live my life?"

And so Roy keeps on trying to prove that he's a free man. He rebels: he overeats.

## The Stand-Up Comic ☐

Instead of rebelling against other people's well-intentioned commands, the Stand-Up Comic pretends she's conforming completely to a sensible eating program. But what the Stand-Up Comic does is delude herself. This personality type was suggested by stand-up comic Joan Rivers. Joan's overeating pattern mimics her nightclub and concert performances—she does it all standing up.

"I tell myself if I do the eating while I'm standing up, it doesn't count," Joan explained. "Only food that you eat sitting down at the table counts. That's the food that goes on your hips, that pads your tushie. I wait until my daughter, Melissa, has gone out to play or to school. Then I head right for the refrigerator. Let's see what we've got: some Twinkies, leftover casserole, cheese, lots of good stuff. So I stand there with the refrigerator door wide open, and I eat. Thirty seconds: whoops, there's half a Twinkie gone. Another couple of minutes: good-bye cheese. Whatever's in the refrigerator is fair game."

Joan does have something to control her stand-up binges —her dogs. "The minute I start eating, the dogs come out from nowhere and they look up at me with those big, brown eyes, so I have to feed them. Otherwise, I'd be the Goodyear blimp by now."

Actually, Joan keeps herself quite trim. She eats with great restraint—when she's sitting down. "If I've eaten too much for breakfast or lunch that day and we have a dinner appointment, I will just sit there for the whole meal and not eat—well, hardly eat anything. I know I have to atone for the calories I already ate."

And if there were excess calories, Joan probably acquired them standing up, fooling herself that as long as you remain on your feet, calories don't count—they just go marching away on foot.

## The Plague of Locusts ☐

One of the most dreaded plagues, from biblical times to the present, has been the horde of locusts. They descend on a field full of grain and devour every edible item in sight, until all the poor farmer has left to show for his labors is a bunch of twigs stripped clean of vegetation. When God really wanted to punish the Egyptians for not letting Moses take the Israelites out of Egypt, He sent them a plague of locusts. In other words, a plague of locusts is to be feared, dreaded, and generally abhorred.

Unfortunately, some of the nicest people you will meet turn into one-person Plagues of Locusts when they overeat. If his personality pattern dictates this kind of overeating behavior, this poor soul will eat virtually anything that isn't nailed down. Whatever's on the table, in the refrigerator, in the pantry—it all goes. Vroom, vroom, the Plague of Locusts overeater devours any food within striking distance. He functions like a human threshing machine; the food just disappears into the nervously chomping maw.

Plague of Locusts eating is usually triggered by severe stress, since this is a rather drastic form of overeating behavior.

Marcia's mother had been hospitalized for a suspected heart attack. Meanwhile, Marcia was trying to carry on as usual with her kids and her home life. It was her work as a den mother that led to Marcia's worst Plague of Locusts episode: "I had ordered twelve dozen doughnuts for a Cub Scout outing. I went to pick them up in my car. When I got all those doughnuts home, I just went berserk. I was so worried about my mother's condition that I didn't know what I was doing. Before I knew it, I had eaten all the doughnuts! Can you believe that? I ate every doughnut in sight. It was so embarrassing. There I was with all those empty doughnut cartons and the worst case of the heaves you could imagine, and I'm supposed to go out and behave like Mrs. Perfect All-American Den Mother that afternoon? Forget it."

Sometimes the Plague of Locusts behavior pattern is a one-time-only situation. But for other people, the Plague of Locusts syndrome is their unavoidable way of life. If they see food, they'll eat it—all of it. Besides the unwanted calories and the accompanying unwanted fat, the Plague of Locusts behavior pattern can drive the overeater to despair, as it escalates the food bills—up and up and up.

## The Broken Dam ☐

This common overeating personality emerges suddenly in a previously well-controlled eater; this syndrome can take over a person's life for years at a time. It's as if a dam of self-control has broken down. And the flood waters—in this case, floods of food—pour in, obliterating whatever traces remain of the dam.

To many people, the Broken Dam personality is just an extreme example of "letting go." After years of conscious food deprivation and steady dieting to maintain a trim shape, the Broken Dam overeater will just give up the effort and let go. This usually occurs when a long-sought goal associated with thinness has been reached.

For many men and women, the Broken Dam personality emerges after marriage: "I starved for ten years to catch a good mate, so now that I've got that marriage license and this wedding ring, I'm going to eat to make up for everything I denied myself in my spouse-hunting years."

It's not just achieving a life goal that can trigger the Broken Dam syndrome. A severe trauma can also unhinge a formerly controlled eater. Mark remembers that his divorce started him off on the Broken Dam syndrome: "After we split up, I didn't have to listen to her constant nagging about keeping my stomach flat. I didn't have to please anybody anymore except myself. So I ate. I ate to make up for all those years I'd suppressed my appetite so that I could look good for her."

A major change in life-style can disrupt eating habits as well, and thus lead to the Broken Dam pattern. Janet always had "a lovely figure," until she became pregnant with her first child. Janet had wanted to be slim to attract and keep her husband, but once she became pregnant her whole way of life altered. She quit work and concentrated on motherhood and the baby. During her pregnancy, Janet had the excuse to eat for literally two—or three or four or more. In her case, the dam of self-control had ruptured almost completely. Janet put on forty pounds before the baby arrived.

After she took the child home from the hospital, Janet made a sincere effort to reduce, but she didn't realize that her basic eating pattern had become the Broken Dam lifestyle. She ate whatever and whenever she wanted, and then would berate herself for her lack of willpower and self-control.

Janet could not succeed at dieting because she was treating only the symptoms (fat) and not the cause. She had achieved her life's major long-term goals—marriage and motherhood—and subconsciously the need to remain slimly attractive no longer exerted a compelling force upon her eating habits. The dam had broken, and excess calories fairly flooded Janet's physical system. She had let go in a big way. Big in every sense of the word.

**The Depression Baby** ☐

Look inside your kitchen cupboards, your refrigerator, your freezer. Are these storage spaces full, empty, or stocked with just what you've planned to consume during the next week or so? A lot can be understood about your basic eating syndrome if you examine the contents of your food-storage areas. For the moment, the kind of food is less important than the quantity of food you find stashed away.

Is food crammed into every cupboard shelf? Is your refrigerator bulging with so much food that something's going to rot before even an overeating family can get around to consuming it? If you serve tomato soup once a week, do you find that you have five or six or maybe even a dozen cans of tomato soup, standing there in neat rows—"just in case"? Just in case of what?

If you're not expecting guests or a horde of ravenous adolescents in the next few days, it may be difficult for you to answer the question of why there are such vast quantities of food lurking in your kitchen storage space. You yourself may be baffled as to your real reasons for stockpiling so much food: "That's just how I keep house." But actually, these overfull shelves are symptomatic of another common overeating disorder: the Depression Baby syndrome.

108

People in the Depression Baby grouping are particularly concerned, even obsessed, with making sure there's "enough" food in the house at all times. But in their cases, "enough" means far more food than they can reasonably eat in the near future. Their pantries may even look like the stockpiles of staple food items that people used to keep in nuclear fallout shelters in the fifties. And that's a *lot* of food!

The food isn't necessarily on the Depression Baby's shelves to be eaten. It's the *presence* of the food itself that is crucial to the Depression Baby, because these food stockpiles impart symbolic security and safety.

The Depression Baby personality type is so widespread that it has categories. These subgroups are defined by what causes this obsessive collecting and storing—and, ultimately, eating—of food. The first variety of Depression Baby is typified by Lucia, a mildly overweight woman in her fifties. Lucia's family was dirt-poor during the Depression. "A lot of the time there wasn't enough food on the table at home," she recalls. "My mother could make a pound of ground meat serve six people for three meals. She mixed it with bread crumbs, with pasta, with anything that was filling and cheap. I can't really say I went to bed hungry too many times during my growing-up years, but there was constant worry about how we were going to put food on the table."

Lucia remembers how her mother would go hungry to leave more food for her children: "It was my mother who usually ate the least. That way we children could get enough nourishment. And the food we did get was not the best—day-old bread, overripe fruits and vegetables, canned goods in dented tins that had been reduced."

When she grew up and had a home of her own, Lucia was obsessive about keeping a well-stocked larder. The idea of running out of a food staple makes her vaguely uneasy. "I make sure to have extras of every item I cook, just so there'll be enough. The minute I'm down to three cans of tuna fish, let's say, I run out to the store and get three more cans." It doesn't matter much to Lucia if those cans sit on her shelves and gather dust for months, even years. The mere presence of the cans and boxes makes her feel there's an underlying stability to her placid, middle-class existence.

When she gets really nervous, Lucia succumbs to stockpiling food in another way—by overeating. She eats vast quantities of pasta, of baked goods, of the freshest and most expensive vegetables and fruits. It's her way of proving to herself that the food won't run out unexpectedly. She stockpiles the food not only on her shelves but inside her body. And to this day, Lucia has never really connected her Depression Baby need to stockpile food on her pantry and refrigerator shelves with her intermittent need to overeat, to overconsume calories.

"I can't tell you, not to save my soul, why I binge sometimes, why all the best intentions in the world don't work on diets," Lucia confesses, puzzled and ashamed of her overeating lapses.

While Lucia's Depression Baby syndrome has its roots in her impoverished childhood, not all Depression Baby stockpilers and overeaters share this background. Some Depression Babies come from firmly middle-class or even wealthy homes. But material possessions could not, for some reason, compensate for a lack of emotional security or for low self-esteem. These Depression Babies are wracked by strong feelings of inner deprivation. That's why they collect food the way other people collect stamps or rare coins. The foods —comfort-related items such as sweets and starches, in particular—give these Depression Babies at least a fleeting sense of well-being.

Wayne was just such a type of Depression Baby. He came from a well-to-do family, so there was no actual lack of food in his case, unlike Lucia's. But Wayne's father was a harsh and unsympathetic man, an arbitrary disciplinarian. "No matter how much I strived to achieve in school, in the Scouts, on high school and college teams, my father never did have a good word for me," Wayne remembers. "Nothing I did was ever good enough to satisfy him." As a result, Wayne, as a grown man, still felt inadequate, because he had never won his father's love.

It was fruitless to try to obtain his father's caring and support, but Wayne could find another way of overcoming his feelings of emotional deprivation: he could stockpile food. Food, to Wayne, subconsciously symbolized a whole range of emotional warmth, of emotional supports. By collecting gourmet delicacies and amassing more fresh fruits and vegetables than he and his family could possibly eat before they spoiled, Wayne was trying to compensate for feeling unloved and worthless.

"I never made the connection between stocking up on food and my problems relating to my dad until one day when I opened up the refrigerator," Wayne said. "Food actually spilled out of the fridge and landed on the floor. I had bought so much food, my wife couldn't fit it all inside the refrigerator and the freezer in the basement. She had always told me I overbought food, but I would just tell her I didn't believe in skimping on necessities.

"But that day when food plopped on the kitchen floor, it suddenly all clicked. I said to myself, 'Boy, you must really feel deprived to need all this food to shore up your emotions.' Once I connected my overbuying and overeating food with Father's cold behavior toward me, I felt free for the first time in years. I knew why I overate, and gradually I was able to cut down on my overeating and lose weight. I would just tell myself, 'You don't need food to substitute for the love you didn't get when you were a child.' "

**The Scavenger** ☐

The seeming opposite of the Depression Baby is the Scavenger overeating pattern. Depression Babies have to conspicuously collect, display, and consume large amounts of food. Underneath it all, Scavenger eaters don't believe they deserve to have food of their own, so they eat other people's food, a nibble at a time. Some Scavengers grew up as poor relations, and this feeling persists into their adult lives. Since they feel they're "not as good as other people," they subconsciously don't believe they deserve to have a lot of food on their shelves or on their plates.

Other Scavengers are avid dieters, who pride themselves on their self-control. When they sit down to a family meal, the Scavenger's plate will be ostentatiously low-calorie: cottage cheese, lettuce, white tuna packed in water and served *sans* mayonnaise. If you just looked at their dinner plates, these Scavengers would seem to be martyrs to the cause of weight control and proper eating habits.

But just observe the Scavenger as he or she pounces on high-calorie goodies on other family members' plates. "Gee, that baked potato with cream cheese and bacon bits looks yummy," the Scavenger whines piteously. "Mind if I take a teeny taste?" The "teeny taste" may very likely turn into half of that "yummy" baked potato. Or else the Scavenger may wind up begging enough "tiny nibbles" of chocolate layer cake (a couple of "tiny nibbles" from each family member's plate) to add up to a couple of pieces. While seemingly dietetically virtuous, the Scavenger is toting up hundreds, even thousands, of extra calories from the plates of spouse, children, even guests. It's a kind of near-invisible overeating, since the Scavenger seldom fills his own plate. And then comes the Scavenger's familiar refrain, "I don't know how I put on those five pounds. Just look—there's nothing on my plate, nothing."

"I'll just pick" is another favorite Scavenger phrase. Playwright Albert Innaurato hilariously captured the Scavenger's overeating tricks in the character of the skinny widow, Lucille Pompi, from his long-running Broadway comedy *Gemini*. At a party feast Lucille leaves her own plate empty. "I'm not really hungry," she sighs. "I'll just pick."

Familiar words—everyone has a friend or relative who utters those same memorable words. But the way Lucille "picks" is comedically bizarre. By the end of the party meal scene in *Gemini,* she has devoured a plateful of spaghetti (compiled from several guests' plates), a load of antipasto, and also the odd meatball. She isn't hungry, she'll just pick, but Lucille winds up guzzling enough food to sustain two brawny stevedores all by her skinny little overeating self.

## The Taster ☐

The Scavenger eats food from other people's plates or surreptitiously chugs down other people's leftovers. But the Taster is another kind of Scavenger: an early bird who gets the worm (or the wurst). It's one of the most insidious overeating patterns, because the Taster syndrome emerges without any kind of underlying neurosis or trauma to blame it on.

The Taster pattern arises out of simple absentmindedness as you cook and prepare food for yourself and others. In fact, the Taster is a classic overeating pattern for women, particularly housewives, since women are usually the ones responsible for family cooking.

Denise is just such a Taster. She's in her forties, the mother of three, not too overweight, but those excess pounds all seem to be clustered in one unsightly zone. "If I don't wear a girdle," she jokes, "my stomach ends up sitting on my thighs." Denise loves to cook, and as she cooks substantial repasts for her clan, she tastes the food. She tastes to see if there's enough salt, tastes to see if there's enough sugar or pepper or tarragon. "Is it done? Is it overcooked?" Well, how else is Denise supposed to tell if the food she's so lovingly prepared tastes good enough to serve to her family and guests unless she tastes it herself?

The question, obviously, is rhetorical. There is no other adequate way, really, for a cook to tell how a particular dish has turned out unless he or she tastes it. Sniffing, prodding with a fork, or simply gazing at a golden crust or whipped egg-white peaks is not sufficient. The proof of the pudding is in the tasting.

And so the Tasters taste. A nibble here, a lick there. And that's why most Tasters are sincerely mystified when extra pounds creep onto their once trim frames. "But I really don't overeat," the Tasters protest. And they're half right. They don't overeat at the dinner table. They just overeat at the stove.

## The TV Diner ☐

TV Diners don't overeat at the dinner table either. Much like the Taster, the TV Diner eats as an accompaniment or aid to another activity. In the TV Diners' cases, it's to accompany their television viewing. Television provokes many people to start stuffing their mouths with junk food, crunchy snacks, and sandwiches hurriedly constructed within the span of a station break or a two-minute segment of commercials.

This habit is so prevalent that it may safely be assumed that the television commercial and the station break are leading causes for the excess of fat in the land. Let's face it, there's very little you can do within a two-minute commercial segment—unless you're one of those strange souls who actually enjoy watching commercials. You can go to the bathroom. You can let out the cat. You can check to see if the kids are sleeping soundly in their beds. Or you can go to the kitchen and whip up a little snack. Like a no-fuss-to-fix bag of potato chips or Fritos, a bowl of ice cream, a peanut-butter-and-jelly sandwich, a handful of Oreo cookies.

It's no accident that the ascendancy of television viewing as a recreation/time-filler was accompanied by the development of the foil-covered, carbohydrate-loaded TV dinner. And where else to eat a TV dinner but in front of a television set?

And as TV dinners proliferated in the fifties and sixties, so did TV Diners. Jed is your common, garden-variety, next-door-neighbor type of TV Diner. "We have one of those little tiny Japanese TV sets in the kitchen, so I usually watch the 'Today' show in the morning while I eat my breakfast. Saves time. You can get two things done at once that way." When he comes home, Jed often nibbles a snack in front of the TV while he watches the network evening news. After dinner, Jed and his family cluster around the TV set once more. A vague, mild boredom sets in. Some additional stimulus is needed besides the TV prime-time programs. Why not food? Out come the junk foods, the crunchy snacks, the after-dinner second desserts.

This kind of TV Diner doesn't even realize what he's shoveling into his system. He's too preoccupied with watching the program to notice very much of what's traveling down his gullet. Watching sports events can be the most calorie-filled time for the chronic TV Diner. Sports events have a built-in anxiety factor, because the fan doesn't know if his favorite team or competitor will win or lose. Consider the average American home on Super Bowl Sunday—six-packs of beer, chips, popcorn, hamburgers or hot dogs, onion rings, maybe a pizza. That one Super Bowl game can put a good three or four pounds of fresh avoirdupois onto a chronic TV Diner.

"The worst part about eating in front of the television is that you don't really notice that you're eating," Jed comments. "Somehow or other, you just *consume* the food, without noticing if it's good or not, or if you're hungry or not. It gets to be a really hard habit to break. I've tried, so I know. If I sit in front of the television set for an hour or two, I get this uneasy feeling. Something's missing if I don't have a snack. You can actually get antsy, trying to overcome that mindless urge to eat and watch prime-time shows simultaneously. You see, watching TV alone wasn't satisfying to me. I had to eat *and* watch TV to feel satisfied."

Because he understands his own particular overeating pattern, Jed has devised a simple yet effective way to diet: "If I want to lose a few pounds, I just have to give up watching TV for a week or two. Then it's amazing how the weight just rolls off. When I watch TV in the evenings, I almost always have at least a bagful of Doritos—that's my favorite. Well, a bag of Doritos has almost a thousand calories. Just give that up for a week, and theoretically, I've lost two pounds right off the bat."

In other words, if you're a perpetual TV Diner, reach for the off button on the TV set, if you expect your weight-control regime to succeed.

## The Grand Prix Nosher ☐

As we've seen, for many people it's not the amount of food consumed at regular meals that puts on the pounds, it's the haphazard consumption of snacks and other unnecessary calories that can transform a flat stomach into a pot belly. The Grand Prix Nosher, much like the TV Diner, uses eating as an accompaniment to another activity. In the case of the Grand Prix Nosher, that activity is driving. These people love to drive, and what's more, they love to eat while they drive. Some people with really severe fixations on Grand Prix Noshing have literally turned their cars into mobile dining rooms.

Actually, it's quite logical to mesh eating and driving in a combined behavior pattern. Driving is the perfect form of escape—drive away from your family, your job, your debts, your loneliness. Any conflict or problem can be driven away from. And that's how many people use their cars— less as a means of transportation than as a means of escape. Similarly, overeating is very often used as a means of escape. The action of eating, in effect, blocks out unpleasant or unwanted thoughts. The action of eating makes you feel as if you're doing something, not just sitting idly. Thus, eating can also serve as an escape from admitting your own inertia.

The Grand Prix Nosher style of overeating can occur in any age group. But it's particularly common among teenagers and young adults. For them, driving a car still has some degree of novelty. In fact, the hours they spend behind the wheel may be the only time they feel free, utterly free, from the constraints of parents, teachers, bosses, and other authority figures.

Don became a Grand Prix Nosher when he was sixteen— the year he got his driver's license. "After school, a few buddies would hop into my car, and we'd drive for a while, maybe stop at a hamburger stand or a pizzeria. We'd take the food out into the car and eat it there. It made us feel grown-up or something, that we had wheels, and we could go where we wanted when we wanted. I ate in the car a lot, so I began to associate the freedom I got from driving with freedom through noshing, too."

When he and his parents would have a spat, Don would storm out of the house, rev up his car, and tear out, bound not for glory but for Burger King. He drove away out of rebellion and ate in the car out of rebellion, too. "My senior year in high school, I started eating breakfast in the car, too. I'd go to McDonald's, buy an Egg McMuffin and some coffee, and gobble it down while I drove."

Grand Prix Noshing lends itself to fast-food places, to cruising down those long stretches of suburban roads that are lined with fast-food franchises, with McDonald's cheek to jowl against Colonel Sanders's Kentucky Fried Chicken next to Arthur Treacher's Fish and Chips. A really dedicated Grand Prix Nosher will make a slow, stately, calorie-filled procession, pulling in and out of one franchise after another, until satiety or nausea or empty wallet occurs.

After a while, a Grand Prix Nosher may actually feel awkward sitting down at a table with real silverware. He has come to associate pleasurable eating with resting paper plates on steering wheels or wedging cola cans between the upholstery and the gear shift on the floor. Since trains are generally passé in this country, today's dining car may be just that—a car in which a Grand Prix Nosher is swiftly, thoughtlessly stuffing his face.

### The World Traveler ☐

As we've already noted, overeating serves as a relatively easy-to-come-by means of escape for many people. The World Traveler takes that notion of escape and goes one step further with it. It's the content of the food he eats that creates the illusion of escape, not merely the act of (over)-eating.

Robert is the World Traveler sort of overeater. He reports that he'll generally overeat when no one else is around, and then he'll eat rapidly "as if calorie count is somehow tied to elapsed eating time." But Robert's moods are crucial to his World Traveler eating pattern: "There is the Italian mood, which only pizza can satisfy. There is the Chinese mood, which only a New York–style eggroll can deal with. Alas, nothing like a New York–style eggroll exists in Los Angeles, where I now live, so often crude substitutes like frozen egg rolls have to suffice. And then there's the Mexican mood, when only tacos or burritos will do the trick."

Even Robert himself can't predict when one of these World Traveler eating "moods" will strike. But he has noticed over the years that "these moods generally make their presence known after a normally stomach-filling dinner which is usually not one of the above types of food. After dinner, I sit around the house and feel bored or frustrated or maybe even trapped. I don't know exactly, but all of a sudden I just want to eat some kind of ethnic delicacy. It seems then that that's the only thing that'll bring me up out of this blue funk."

Without consciously realizing it, Robert has made food his way of escaping from his mundane, workaday life. If he can't pull up stakes and leave his house and job and spouse in Los Angeles, then Robert can at least take a gastronomic journey—if not through the canals of Venice or Amsterdam or Bangkok, then at least through the canals of his own gastrointestinal tract.

### The Clock Watcher ☐

This overeating type cares more about what the hands of a clock say than what his body says to him. He eats when the clock informs him, "Now's the time to be hungry," instead of when he actually feels hunger pangs.

The Clock Watcher tends to be easily influenced by family and peers in regard to his eating behavior. It's an eating style that has its origins far back in childhood, when parents told the child when it was time to eat. And whether he was hungry or not, the child was expected to "eat all those peas and carrots off that plate or you won't get any dessert." So it's no wonder that so many people fall victim to the Clock Watcher syndrome; it's been indoctrinated in their minds for most of their lives.

"When I was growing up, we sat down to dinner at 6:00 P.M. on the dot, and I must have learned to sit down and eat then, no matter what, just like one of Pavlov's dogs, salivating as it were, when I saw the hands of the clock strike six," recalls Nancy, a confirmed Clock Watcher.

This habit persisted into Nancy's adult life. If she saw that 6:00 P.M. was approaching, and dinner wasn't ready, she'd feel vaguely anxious—and hungry. She might eat a meal at six o'clock before going out to a dinner party, where she knew she might not eat until after eight o'clock. Like many Clock Watchers, Nancy learned to disregard her body's inner signals about hunger and satiety. When it turned six o'clock, she assumed she felt hungry. Actually, she didn't "consult" her stomach at all—she just ate because the time was "right."

Stanley Schachter, the Columbia University psychologist who conducted many noted obesity research experiments, tested the Clock Watchers syndrome scientifically in 1968. With his associate Larry P. Gross, Schachter constructed an experiment using a doctored clock, a clock that would run at either twice the normal speed or half the normal speed. The hypothesis: that obese experimental subjects would depend on the clock's time (an external stimulus) to tell them when they felt hungry, rather than relying on their own physiological signs of hunger or satiety (internal stimuli) to tell them whether to eat or not. Schachter and Gross believed that overweight subjects would consume more of the snack crackers they were offered when their incorrect clocks in the experimental room showed that it was dinner time.

The results of the experiment were striking and amply proved the experimenters' hypothesis. Overweight experimental subjects ate *twice* as many crackers when shown a clock that read closer to mealtimes than did overweight subjects whose clocks read farther from mealtimes. Normal-weight subjects weren't much affected by what the doctored clocks said—they ate the proffered crackers when they felt hungry, not when the clock told them to eat.

In other words, Schachter and Gross experimentally showed that people with weight problems (their overweight subjects) disregarded their bodies' internal eating cues (hunger) and relied instead on an arbitrary external cue (the false clocks) to tell them whether or not to eat.

The experiment proved that the Clock Watcher overeating pattern does exist. That's small comfort to Clock Watchers like Nancy, who knew very well that this problem existed with or without benefit of documented scientific evidence. Life has taught Nancy that the Clock Watcher syndrome is a very real, hard-to-eradicate overeating problem. And Nancy didn't need doctored clocks or piles of experimental snack crackers to prove it. All she needed was her own drive (impelled by clock hunger) toward the stove or refrigerator when six o'clock rolled around.

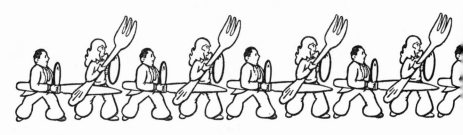

# 8  Eating Personalities: Overeaters, II

Overeating is so prevalent that covering the various overeating personality types requires two chapters. Here are fifteen more overeating personality types, whose origins range from cultural conditioning and situational responses to emotional compensation and acting out.

Remember to keep on jotting down your ten-point scale evaluation numbers next to each new overeating type. That way, by the time you finish reading these two chapters on overeaters, you won't just recognize overeating in others; you'll be able to recognize the *specific* overeating dimensions in your own personality.

Now, on with the overeaters!

**The Seeker** ☐

Historically, seekers have searched for truth, for enlightenment, for spirituality and peace of mind. But another kind of seeker may be more numerous and just as dedicated as the religious variety. These are the people who are on a perpetual quest to find *some* food that will finally satisfy them, that will finally bring a binge to a stop or an uncontrolled eating life-style under control.

Peggy got into the Seeker eating pattern accidentally. She thought she was reaching an enlightenment about her obsessive relationship to food. Instead, she was entering another, deeper food pitfall.

"I had been on every diet known to man over the years," Peggy confesses. "On and off diets, my weight going up and down. I got very tired of always veering between feast and famine, so I decided to sit down and analyze *why* I would overeat. I came to the conclusion that the foods I was currently eating weren't satisfying me. No matter how much I ate of them, I always felt empty or cheated or that I was getting second-best. I figured, if I can just find something that is really delicious, it'll satisfy me, and then I won't want to overeat anymore."

And that's how Peggy turned into a Seeker. It was like opening Pandora's Box, and it brought Peggy just about as many woes. "It wasn't enough merely to indulge in ice cream. Now I had to find the best ice cream. So I'd sample this brand, that brand, this flavor, that flavor. Was it better slightly mushy or rock-hard?" In her never-ending quest for the ideal ice cream, Peggy ended up consuming more ice cream than she had when she was content to just gorge briefly on whatever ice cream was available and then flagellate herself with guilt and new promises to herself to resume a sensible diet.

A Seeker often thinks that finding the ideal food will result not in further eating but in blessed satiety—at last. "As long as I'm going off my diet, I should have the best," their reasoning goes. Let's say a Seeker like Peggy goes off her diet because of a yearning for bread. A couple of slices of bread and butter won't do for the Seeker. A survey of available breads is likely to ensue. One day the Seeker will try out pumpernickel, the next day rye, the next day white baked by XYZ Bakery, the day after that white baked by ABC Bakery. The perfect bread is seldom discovered, so the overeating can continue unabated.

The Seeker has set himself an almost impossible task. It is the overeater's equivalent of setting out on a Quest for the Holy Grail. Unless you're Sir Galahad, you have no chance of winning at the Seeker's game. Or as Pete Townshend wrote of religiously inspired seekers in his song "The Seeker": "I won't get to get what I'm after—till the day I die." For eating Seekers, that pretty well sums up their future.

## The Overdoser ☐

The Overdoser operates on an eating principle somewhat similar to the Seeker's. The difference between these two overeating types is that the Overdoser has pinpointed just what foods drive him to excess, to overeat. Now that the Overdoser knows precisely what food turns him on, he wishes he could be turned off—for once and for all. The Overdoser feels his overeating problem will be solved if only he can lose the craving for those particular, special foods.

The Overdoser then decides that the solution to his overeating problem is to overdose himself on those foods until the very sight of them will fill him with revulsion. In other words, he wants to OD on his particular eating vice, be it french fries or Hostess Twinkies.

Bill decided to perform the Overdoser "cure" on himself: "I had this obsession with chocolate-flavored frozen custard cones. I could pack them away like there was no tomorrow, and I could see where those cones were going—right into the paunch I never used to have before. So I decided to go to the Dairy Queen and order the biggest chocolate soft custard cone they made and eat that cone and then another one just as big and then another one, until I couldn't even stand to *look* at a chocolate Dairy Queen cone."

Bill parked his car outside the local Dairy Queen and set about OD-ing on frozen custard cones. He made it through three enormous cones—on top of a full dinner—before the OD effect set in: "Let me tell you, I puked all over that Dairy Queen parking lot. I was sick to my stomach. To this day, I never want to see another chocolate Dairy Queen cone again."

Apparently, the self-inflicted aversion therapy worked. However, it didn't work perfectly. Shortly after his valiant effort in combating his lust for Dairy Queen custard, Bill quite inadvertently developed a fixation on pepperoni pizza. The Overdoser plan of action was implemented again. Presto, no yen for pepperoni pizza beset Bill any longer. Now, however, it was jelly doughnuts that became the objects of his eating passions.

The Overdoser attempts to counteract feelings of deprivation by an overabundance of riches. But even an embarrassment of edible riches—like Bill's multiple gigantic custard cones—doesn't mean this personality type will be "cured" of the desire to overeat. It's not the single kind of food that causes overeating or overweight. It's the basic compulsive desire to eat food that's at the root of the problem and at the root of the Overdoser syndrome. The basic lesson most Overdosers must learn: Enough is never enough. At least, not when it comes to food.

### The Condemned Man ☐

Mankind's fixation on food, particularly on delicacies and abundance, is expressed in many ways in human culture. One example is the condemned man and his last meal. Traditionally (in the West at least), the person condemned to execution has been allowed the privilege of ordering a sumptuous last meal. This was done as a courtesy to the person who was about to die. But it was also another, subtle way of expressing the high value society places on food and on eating well. A filet mignon the night before the execution was supposed to compensate somehow for the fact that the prisoner was going to stand up in front of a firing squad at dawn the next day. Well, the filet mignon may have been delicious, but the condemned man would much rather live.

In just the same way, people who exemplify the Condemned Man eating personality are eating well today to compensate themselves for what they will suffer tomorrow. But Condemned Man eaters aren't going to die tomorrow.

They are merely going to diet. And to many people, dieting is about as pleasant a prospect as going before that firing squad at dawn.

Nearly everyone has indulged in the Condemned Man behavior pattern at some time in his life. Gerri is determined to go on a diet, starting on Monday morning. "A new week, a new start," she reasons. Of course, Gerri has made this decision on Friday evening when she discovers that her slim-cut French jeans fit so snugly that she can barely bend the material enough to sit down, much less to bend over. Heaven forbid! She might have to buy a bigger size.

Gerri resolves to go on a stringent diet . . . starting Monday. So Friday night, she has a gooey dessert and a box of buttered popcorn. "What's the difference? It won't hurt. I'm going on a diet Monday anyhow." Saturday she has a pizza, some rolls, and a Good Humor ice-cream bar. "It won't hurt. I'm going on a diet Monday, for Chrissakes."

Sunday comes along and Gerri is already feeling severe food deprivation, before she's even eaten her first diet meal of hard-boiled eggs, low-fat cottage cheese, and melba toast. She is in a quiet gustatory frenzy. She rifles through her pantry and freezer shelves, seeking any items that will be forbidden to her on the weeks ahead during her diet. She gobbles up everything she fears she might miss, once the diet (the execution, as it were) commences the next day.

Monday Gerri goes on her diet. She is strict with herself. She follows it to the letter. But somehow she's gained three or four more pounds between the time she decided her French jeans were too tight and the time she stepped on the bathroom scale Monday morning.

Like most Condemned Man eaters, Gerri feared the execution of her sentence ("You must go on a strict diet"). She feared this so much that she ate not one but many "last meals." And last meals tend to be heavy in calories, and hence tend to add on more pounds before the diet even begins.

The Condemned Man eater may have fantastic willpower

once he or she is actually *on* the diet. But in the process of beginning the diet, they overeat even more and thus give themselves a far harder task—more weight to lose.

### The Social Eater ☐

Some people are social drinkers. They'll drink only when they're invited to a party or when they're gathered together with friends or family. They can take it or leave it when it comes to drinking. Unlike alcoholics, social drinkers aren't debilitated by their brief forays into alcohol consumption; they aren't slaves to liquor.

Similarly, some people are Social Eaters. They'll overeat only when they're invited to a party or social occasion or when they're entertaining or when they're in the company of friends and family. Of course, that does add up to a lot of "only when" situations. But the Social Eater doesn't *have* to overeat.

Unlike the true compulsive eater, the Social Eater doesn't consume food in an illogical, self-destructive fashion. The Social Eater, more or less, chooses the times he or she intends to overindulge in food. After all, when the food's right there, set out so attractively on the buffet tables, and everybody else is filling his plate, how can you refuse? Well, why not try a little? Just this one time.

The Social Eater is a lot like the Clock Watcher; both allow external stimuli to dictate their eating habits. The Clock Watcher lets the clock tell him the appropriate time to eat. The Social Eater lets other people tell him the appropriate time *and* amount to eat. Social Eaters, you see, are unusually susceptible to peer pressure.

The Social Eater personality has its roots in childhood. Children are taught to associate good manners with partaking of the food their hosts provide—no matter how distasteful that food might be to the potential Social Eater. Mother says, "I know you don't like white cake, but if you don't eat a piece of Johnny's birthday cake, you'll make him feel bad." So a slice of Johnny's birthday cake is dutifully consumed. It's an extension of the childhood training of "Clean your plate, so Mommy and Daddy will be proud of you. Oh, what a good eater you are!"

In the teenage years, the Social Eater may not feel hungry, but he or she wants to be accepted, so if everybody else is going out for fried onion rings and Cokes after the football game, the Social Eater will go along and conform by eating a suitable number of onion rings and swilling a suitable amount of Coke. To fit in with the crowd—that's the point.

By adulthood, the Social Eater pattern of behavior is so deeply instilled that the Social Eater himself doesn't even realize that's why he or she eats. In fact, the adult Social Eater may look forward to parties, dinners, and other social events, where he *has* to eat in order to "be polite" and to conform. Then good manners and peer pressure can be used to the adult Social Eater's advantage: the social occasion becomes a license to eat, drink, and otherwise do a pretty convincing imitation of a pig.

Social Eaters, in a way, represent an almost benign form of overeating personality. Although they don't realize it fully, they *are* in control of their overeating. Once the Social Eater understands why he overeats when he does—that this overeating is not a random, inexplicable occurrence but does have roots and causes—then he can stamp out this kind of overeating fairly easily.

The danger for the Social Eater is parallel to the danger faced by the social drinker. The social drinker can slip over the boundary into alcoholism, in some instances. Similarly, the Social Eater can, in some cases, slip over the boundaries into the more addictive and compulsive forms of overeating.

### The Gourmet Glutton ☐

Being a gourmet is socially acceptable. Being a glutton is not. To camouflage their gluttony—their voracious over-eating—some people pretend to be true gourmets, true con-noisseurs of the finest of food and drink.

While the true gourmet will rarely stuff himself, the Gourmet Glutton eats with all the finesse and selectivity of a McCormick reaper. The jaws open, crunch, swallow, gulp, and the food disappears down the toothy cavity. Much like the shark in *Jaws*, the Gourmet Glutton at times seems to be all enormous mouth and insatiable appetite attached to a vast and mindless hunger.

The Gourmet Glutton is a compulsive overeater like any other, but he tries to infiltrate the more respectable ranks of the food connoisseurs, most of whom would be appalled by the Gourmet Glutton's rapacious appetite and lack of selectivity. A true gourmet chooses his food carefully, eats it slowly while considering the taste sensations aroused, and can knowledgeably discourse about the origins of a particular dish—what ingredients and preparation techniques separate a "merely good" dish from a "superb" one. A true gourmet is practicing a hobby; some might even say practicing the gustatory art form. A Gourmet Glutton is merely practicing a compulsion.

The Gourmet Glutton typically hasn't taken all the time and effort that a gourmet does with his dining. He merely labels himself a gourmet: "Only the best. I eat only the best. If you eat only top-notch stuff, how could you possibly do yourself harm by overeating?"

Real gourmets are appalled by the Gourmet Glutton. Supermarkets and snooty restaurants are enriched by him. And the mere thought of the Gourmet Glutton would have a true food connoisseur like Brillat-Savarin spinning in his grave.

### The One-Food Samba ☐

This overeating personality is akin to both the Seeker and the Overdoser. All are searching for the ideal food: the perfect croissant, the most scrumptious strawberry shortcake, the most luscious pâté de fois gras. But the Seeker is still only seeking, and the Overdoser is trying to sicken himself, while the person doing the One-Food Samba has reached a kind of contentment by finding his perfect food, his ideal treat, his culinary heaven on earth.

This syndrome is not at all uncommon. In fact, it's a rare person who hasn't gone through a period when the One-Food Samba was the song that played continually in his mind. Even the mildest emotional overeater can come across one food that makes him rise to the heights of gustatory passion and desire—the food of the Ultimate Yen. This food monomania might be centered on bagels or on Famous Amos chocolate-chip cookies or even on something fairly nutritious like artichoke hearts or Granny Smith apples.

The precise food of the Ultimate Yen is not really what matters here. But the craving for that food is what matters. The person dancing the One-Food Samba through life has simply *got* to quench this craving—preferably by massive ingestion of the beloved food item. Or he goes very quietly, very specifically berserk.

Ted is a One-Food Samba person who has a craving for bagels. With Ted, it's more than a craving; it's a love affair. Ted loves bagels. He reels as he sniffs a fresh-baked pumpernickel bagel. An onion bagel sends him into giddy waves of ecstasy. And a sesame bagel—to die for. Ted's passionate desire for bagels is a *cri de coeur*—a hunger emanating from deep within the soul and the gastrointestinal cavity.

Part of Ted's love affair with bagels stems from bagels' unavailability in his locale. The difficulty in linking up with his beloved (i.e., his bagels) only inflames Ted's passions further. But even Ted has a hard time locating a bagel in Peoria at eleven o'clock on a Sunday evening. A fresh-baked bagel is not to be found. Ted paces the floor, thinking about bagels hot from the oven. He rolls visions of bagels through his mind, tasting them mentally with his forlorn taste buds.

Still, Ted's first chance to find a fresh-baked bagel occurs the next afternoon, on his lunch break from work. By then, Ted has overcome his compulsion to consume bagels, bagels, and more bagels. The wild yearning for a bagel has subsided into a merely affectionate feeling toward the lumps of dough with holes in their centers. But having located hot bagels in Peoria, Ted decides to eat a couple anyway—to make up for being "deprived" of his beloved Ultimate Yen food the previous night. Absence makes the heart grow fonder, even if the heart in this case is really a stomach.

People experiencing the One-Food Samba will go to ridiculous lengths to get the desired food. Stars like Elizabeth Taylor and Frank Sinatra have been known to import gallons of chili from Chasen's restaurant in Los Angeles to the far ends of the earth when the need, the urge, the One-Food Samba strikes.

Vicky is one woman who would wildly gyrate to the One-Food Samba when she even *thought* of apple strudel. So she decided to stock up on her Ultimate Yen food at the bakery. Vicky bought large quantities of apple strudel, lovingly wrapped each portion, and carefully stored them in her deep freeze. But she neglected to take into account the defrosting time required to make her frozen pastries more pliable than apple-flavored popsicles.

"One night, late, I had this mad desire for a slice of apple strudel," Vicky sighed. "I had to have a slice of apple strudel with coffee, or I *knew* I would go mad. I'm serious. I think at that point I would have killed—or at least have assaulted—for apple strudel. But then I discovered that all my strudel was frozen solid in the deep freeze. I don't know what possessed me—I must have gone stark staring mad. Because the next thing I knew, I was gnawing and licking and sucking at a frozen slab of strudel. It was so icy cold that the strudel was sticking to my tongue and lips.

"Then my son came in and saw what I was doing. I was so ashamed! It's difficult enough to keep the respect of a fourteen-year-old boy without having him see you foaming at the mouth, standing beside an open deep freeze, sucking on a slice of frozen apple strudel, and washing it down with hot coffee, so your gums won't form icicles. I've got to stop eating like this. Someday."

### The Balloon ☐

Some people's weight goes up and down rather haphazardly, depending on whether or not they can muster enough willpower, self-denial, and bottles of diet soda. The Balloon personality has a body weight that veers from hefty highs to svelte lows, but the Balloon can accomplish feats of slenderizing in response to special occasions. The Balloon person is usually inflated with fat, but they can deflate themselves when social and business circumstances demand slimness.

Balloons genuinely love to eat, and they can quite happily allow themselves to get flabby, get a spare tire around the midsection, even get rotund. But give a Balloon a good *reason* to reduce—particularly a special event where he needs to be thin—and the Balloon will become rigorously anti-eating, anti-food, and anti-calories. The Balloon will even starve willingly to crash-deflate his balloonlike figure.

Meg had let herself go. Her figure had swelled to what is politely called "matronly proportions." She might seem a perfect example of the Letting Go/Broken Dam syndrome. But then Meg receives an announcement of her tenth college reunion. Almost miraculously, her appetite disappears, the pounds roll off, her husband is amazed and pleased. By the time the tenth reunion rolls around, Meg looks great again in a size 9.

"It was worth it all, just to see the looks on some of those guys' faces." Meg grinned. "I didn't want them to look at me and then go home, saying, 'Poor old Meg, she really went to seed.' "

After the tenth-reunion dinner-dance, Meg and her spouse went home, and Meg began to eat and overeat once more. "I don't understand it. Why is she doing this to herself again?" Meg's husband moans. "After all the effort she went to to get slim again."

But Meg really has no *reason* to diet now. Her motivation—looking good the night of the tenth-reunion dinner-dance—has passed. By gaining weight again, Meg wasn't reverting to old, bad eating habits. She was just continuing the same cyclical feast-starve syndrome that typifies the true Balloon.

Another classic example of the Balloon personality pattern occurs in the mother of the bride during the three months before the wedding. For most mothers, a daughter's wedding is a big deal. All those relatives you never see except at weddings and funerals now pop up and scurry out from under their rocks. The bride's mother is going to be an integral, albeit sentimentally sobbing, part of the wedding party, and it just wouldn't do to have to confront 150 invited guests while looking like a blimp. So the mother of the bride will, in true Balloon fashion, assiduously diet during those last few months before the marriage festivities. She'll deflate from a size 18 to a size 12—all so that she can look good for the out-of-town guests and for the wedding pictures.

"My God, can you imagine looking like an ox in the wedding pictures and then having to confront that fatso image every time you pull out the family album? Horrors." So the Balloon mother of the bride will slim down. But watch her tuck it in at the wedding dinner. And after the bride and groom are off on their honeymoon, the mother of the bride can return to everyday anonymity. Then she reverts to true form—Balloon form. She goes back to gorging once again.

The most famous celebrity Balloon is undoubtedly Elizabeth Taylor. Taylor loves fattening foods and eating in general. Reportedly, her idea of a good meal is potatoes and beer. Neither item is known for its slimming properties. But Taylor is also a professional, a star. And when she's been scheduled to act in front of the cameras, Taylor has virtually always looked svelte—busty, but svelte. She can apparently deprive herself of excessive food intake when she has a damned good reason—work.

**The Garbage Pail**  ☐

Although these persons may eat to excess, they have basically frugal natures. They simply cannot bear to see good food go to waste. So they feel obligated, duty-bound, even compelled to eat up the leftovers. Instead of throwing food into the garbage pail, people with this eating personality throw food into their mouths. It's more economical. It's also more fattening.

Garbage Pail overeaters aren't a monolithic mass of people who all detest the idea of leftovers. Actually, Garbage Pails fall into two major subgroups.

The more common variety of Garbage Pail is the mother who eats all the food her children leave on their plates. Carla has three small children, and she still "can't get over the amount of food they would waste if I'd let them. You should see all the perfectly good vegetables they leave on their plates. And the amount of green salad they don't even touch. It's a sin, I tell you. You pick up their plates after they've left the table, and there's half a hamburger patty there or a big lump of tuna casserole. I'll bet you could feed an entire family of four in India on the leftovers my three kids leave on their plates. It's disgraceful how much perfectly good, healthy food we Americans waste. Disgraceful."

Carla cleans off her children's plates; then, almost as a patriotic duty, she eats the leftovers. It would be "disgraceful" to let "perfectly good food" go to waste. So Carla chomps away at leftover vegetables, salads, entrées, whatever. She seems to believe it's better for her—or somebody —to eat them, whether she's hungry or not, rather than feeding the leftovers to the garbage disposal.

This is not an intentional overeating pattern, or even a deeply rooted, neurotic overeating syndrome. Carla's overeating pattern is culturally caused. She eats like a Garbage Pail almost unconsciously, having been taught from childhood that she should eat everything on her plate, since "children in Europe are starving."

Almost every twentieth-century American child has undergone this indoctrination of waste not, want not, feeling guilty about the starving foreigners. Generations of children have learned to feel guilty about the starving masses in Europe, Armenia, India, Latin America, Africa, and Southeast Asia. (Take your pick of starving areas, according to your generation.)

And that's why people like Carla dutifully devour their kids' leftovers. "Don't forget, children in Europe are starving." That's what Carla subliminally hears in her head. Well, Carla sure as hell isn't starving; if she keeps on eating à la the Garbage Pail, she'll be bloating instead of wasting away.

Another example of Garbage Pail overeater is the single person who deplores wasting food. This kind of Garbage Pail doesn't have children who waste their food by leaving leftovers. This Garbage Pail is driven by the American food industry's custom of packaging virtually all processed, prepared foods in multiple-unit containers.

Let's say George, a single-person Garbage Pail, has decided to have a chocolate-covered doughnut. All George wants is one chocolate-covered doughnut—just one. But if he decides to buy that doughnut in a supermarket or convenience shop, instead of at a bakery or doughnut fast-food franchise, old George is going to be out of luck. Because of the way food is packaged in most American supermarkets, it's nearly impossible to buy just one chocolate-covered doughnut. The doughnuts come only in boxes of six or twelve.

So George decides to buy a six-pack of doughnuts, even though he wants only one. He sensibly consumes a single doughnut, then puts its sister doughnuts away on a shelf. But all those leftover doughnuts sing a siren call of waste not, want not to George. He realizes that he's got five perfectly good doughnuts on his shelf that will go stale and be no good to anyone, unless George the Garbage Pail polishes them off.

It's a sin to waste food—George has learned his childhood lessons well, so well that he has a knee-jerk reflex toward consuming food, not a well-reasoned response. And George thus winds up eating all six doughnuts. He'll act like a true Garbage Pail, stuffing six doughnuts into his face, when all he originally craved and hungered for was one. Just a little one, at that.

As the plight of the Garbage Pails points out, childhood lessons about eating become so deeply ingrained that they're hard to detect, much less to root out. Food has many deep-seated emotional connotations to most people, and these associations of food with warmth, love, comfort, and well-being are formed early in infancy. That's why at times of stress, particularly at times of homesickness, food often serves as a panacea.

This is how the Home, Home on the Range personality pattern sets in—via homesickness. Grasping for some straw that will reunite him with his home, his loved ones, the person acting out Home, Home on the Range will actively seek out those special foods and delicacies that stand out in his childhood memories.

The old cowboy song "Home, Home on the Range" recalled a mythical Western plain "where seldom was heard a discouraging word." This kind of overeater wants that feeling again, but for him the Home, Home on the Range is more likely to resemble Mama's or Grandma's kitchen range than a flat Texas plain. The person experiencing the Home, Home on the Range behavior pattern wants relief from homesickness and stress. He believes that relief will come through a symbolic form of regression to his childhood or to happier days of the past.

That regression doesn't take the form of thumb-sucking or childish temper tantrums. Instead, that regression takes the form of consuming soothing quantities of ethnic delicacies—pirogi and kielbasa, perhaps, for a Polish-American, pasta for an Italian-American, chicken soup and kishke for a Jewish-American. Or if the Home, Home on the Range person stems from a completely Americanized family, the desired foods may be regional in origin: boiled dinner and Indian pudding for New Englanders, grits and southern fried chicken for southerners, burritos and tostadas for southern Californians.

The food in and of itself doesn't do the soothing, the comforting. It's the long-term good feelings and experiences associated with those foods that cast a spell resulting in the Home, Home on the Range syndrome.

Tracey had always lived near her parents. But when a new job opportunity opened up a thousand miles away from her family's hometown, she couldn't resist taking it. A stranger in a new city, she tried to bury herself in her work. But during the long, often lonely evenings, Tracey would feel tense, anxiety-ridden, and finally homesick. She'd pace around her apartment, filled with nervous energy.

One evening Tracey decided to use that nervous energy, expending it in cooking. Seemingly at random, she decided to make corned beef and cabbage and Irish soda bread— exactly the kinds of foods her favorite, Irish grandmother used to prepare when Tracey went over to visit her on Sunday afternoons as a child. Pretty soon, Tracey was hooked on Irish cooking. Every night she'd busy herself, cooking with a brogue. Her feelings of loneliness, of being adrift away from her loved ones in a strange city, would dissipate for at least the few hours she spent cooking and eating "homey" foods.

Home, Home on the Range produced a partial release from the stress and homesickness of settling in a new town. But Home, Home on the Range also produced a few unexpected bulges on Tracey's hips and thighs. And when she went home for Christmas, her family kept pestering her to take off all that new-formed fat before it "solidified" and became impossible to reduce.

Even athletes—who are constantly concerned with their physical perfection and body performance—can fall prey to overeating personality patterns. Champion tennis player Martina Navratilova was clearly suffering from the Home, Home on the Range pattern after she defected from her native Czechoslovakia to the United States. Although she was playing tournament tennis virtually every week—and there's hardly a better way to burn up calories—Navratilova kept putting on pounds.

136

It turned out that she felt homesick, so she was over-eating. First she overate Czech foods that reminded her of home ("Home, Home on the Range" incarnate); then she overate typically American foods, trying to feel more comfortable, more at home, in this gastronomically strange country. Only when her homesickness subsided could Navratilova lose her Home, Home on the Range pounds and get herself down to truly competitive trim.

## The Fortress of Fat  ☐

People who are enveloped in the Home, Home on the Range syndrome use food as a source of comfort and security. But people who exemplify the Fortress of Fat personality use food as a defense. The overeating itself isn't the payoff for the Fortress of Fat individual. Rather, it's the physical result of overeating—the fat added to the body, the unfashionable, unattractive chunky or heavy appearance—that is their real, though usually unconscious, goal.

Why would anyone *want* to look overweight? In the case of the Fortress of Fat individuals, this personality pattern results from fears about sex, sexuality, and sexual desirability.

Conventional psychoanalytic wisdom has attributed many, if not most, cases of overweight and compulsive eating to fears about sex.

However, more recent psychological research by Dr. Judith Rodin and others have shown that the Fortress of Fat personality and syndrome is *not* typical of overweight people. On the contrary, some studies have said overweight women, in particular, are more highly sexed than their thinner counterparts.

Only a minority of people with weight problems, then, are beset by the Fortress of Fat mentality—so don't let well-meaning but misinformed friends persuade you that the real reason you're not thin is because of a secret fear of sex. 'Tain't so.

Jenny has been a Fortress of Fat for most of her life without ever realizing it. Oh, it's not that Jenny has been heavy all her life. Like many people locked into this eating syndrome, Jenny can get rather thin and stay there—just as long as nobody tells her that she looks good.

Once people begin to tell Jenny how splendidly slim she looks, the Fortress of Fat mentality swings into action. Much to her conscious mind's dismay, Jenny finds that she's on a perpetual eating binge. Her figure is going downhill and her weight is climbing up scale, as her unconscious mind's fears impel her toward an eating binge that lasts until she's "safely" overweight and unattractive again.

You see, the Fortress of Fat person uses excess weight as an excuse for avoiding social contacts and, especially, sexual relationships. Although Jenny has a good job and seems to function normally in the "real" world, she is beset by hidden feelings of inferiority, especially of sexual inferiority.

"My father was constantly putting me down when I was a young girl," she remembers. "He told me that I was a slob, that I was clumsy, that I was hopelessly unfeminine. I tried to shrug off those ideas, but somehow, despite all my efforts to build up my confidence, I always have this lingering doubt about my own attractiveness and desirability as a woman."

As long as she's overweight, and hence unattractive (in her opinion), Jenny feels "safe" on a certain emotional level: she's in no shape (literally) to compete for men's attentions. And since she can't compete, she can't lose. It's as if an athlete with a broken leg is consoling himself by thinking, "I could've won that track meet if it hadn't been for this cast on my leg." Jenny doesn't have a cast on her leg that cripples her chances in the race for men's attentions and affections. But Jenny does have a Fortress of Fat surrounding her body, preventing her from feeling attractive—but also preventing her from failing.

"One time I got really thin—at least, it was really thin for me. Down to 120 pounds. I looked great. I thought every man for miles around would come running, because I was such a sensational-looking woman.

"Well, funny thing—I wasn't much more popular than I was before I lost all the weight. The guys I wanted didn't want me. One man that I thought I had caught, that I thought might even marry me—he dropped me for a girl who was *naturally* thin and gorgeous. I didn't have a chance, even when I looked the best I could look, the thinnest I could get, so I figured why fight it. Might as well eat up and enjoy myself."

Like many people imprisoned in their own Fortresses of Fat, Jenny is afraid to let the opposite sex come close, both literally and figuratively, because that might lead to involvement. And involvement might lead to rejection. Jenny fears that men might realize that she is second-rate in feminine desirability, the message her father had dunned into her head all during her growing-up years.

So for Jenny, being slim and attractive wouldn't lead to a reward. It would, in her mind, lead to ultimate psychological pain, when the men she had attracted by her good figure would see the "inferior woman" that Jenny really was underneath—the inferior woman that her father had convinced her she would be, no matter how she looked.

Thus, men and women locked up in the Fortress of Fat personality avoid the problem of sexual involvement and possible rejection altogether. They hide within their bulging but secure Fortresses of Fat. They use cellulite as body armor. "Look at me—I'm encircled by fat, so nobody can get past my body's fortress and hurt me. Nobody."

One study done by Dr. Albert J. Stunkard, a leading obesity researcher, proved the existence of this Fortress of Fat personality structure. Stunkard gathered information from over seventy psychoanalysts. After analyzing the data, Stunkard found that nearly half of the obese patients seeing this group of psychoanalysts had admitted that they ate too much and grew heavy because they were afraid of sex.

Oddly enough, Stunkard found that most of these obese patients hadn't gone into analysis to lose weight. (Studies by social psychologist I. S. Czarnik show that psychotherapy doesn't usually help most people for long-term weight loss and weight maintenance anyway.) These obese people had consulted their analysts because of symptoms of depression and anxiety. Do the depression and anxiety result from being overweight or does overweight arise from depression and anxiety? That appears to be an unanswerable question —rather like "Which came first, the chicken or the egg?"

For people in the Fortress of Fat, the question isn't very interesting. Not unless you tell them that they look wonderful—so slim, so trim. And then the Fortress of Fat individual will mindlessly, fearfully gobble down both the chicken and the egg, already on his way to developing a coating of fatty body armor, the better to blunt the world's pains.

## The Night Stalker ☐

Vampires aren't the only creatures who feed only at night. So does the Night Stalker type of overeater. The Night Stalker has very little trouble getting through the day in complete control of his eating habits. His food consumption is moderate; he pretty much sticks to the traditional "three squares" a day. But around 2:00 A.M., the Night Stalker arises from his sleep, driven by an insatiable hunger. A vampire would crave blood during his nocturnal hunts for food. But a Night Stalker overeater is more likely to crave a big hunk of that leftover roast in the refrigerator or a huge wedge of cherry pie. His stomach rumbling—or something disturbing in his subconscious that surfaces during dreams —causes the Night Stalker to drag himself wearily from his bed and stagger downstairs to the kitchen, where he somnambulistically raids the fridge, freezer, and pantry.

The Night Stalker's nocturnal forays have been immortalized in many aspects of popular culture. The most famous fictional Night Stalker is undoubtedly Dagwood Bumstead of the "Blondie" cartoon strip. Dagwood sleepwalks into the kitchen in the middle of the night, while Blondie, the kids, and the dogs are sound asleep. Operating more through touch than sight (his eyes are usually shut in the drawings), Dagwood constructs a monumental, multilayered sandwich. These creations gave rise to the Dagwood sandwich found on many diner menus.

After Dagwood gulps down his gargantuan snack, he

peacefully sleepwalks back upstairs to bed. Inevitably, the cartoonist has Dagwood awake the next morning—starving. Dagwood's Night Stalks have caused so much laughter over the decades because his nocturnal overeating behavior strikes a familiar chord. Dagwood is like people we know. Maybe even like ourselves.

Pete is a Night Stalker. He has been for several years, ever since he went into business for himself and started waking up in the middle of the night, "thinking about my books not balancing. I'd be so shook up, I'd have to get out of bed to get the nightmare out of my head. I didn't want to wake up my wife to talk it out, so I'd just step into the kitchen and fix a snack."

Because the Night Stalker's overeating is largely neat and nocturnal, the rest of the family is mystified. Why is Daddy (or Mommy) packing on the pounds when nobody ever sees him/her overeat? And they're also somewhat befuddled, because they can never quite figure out how the fridge can be full at bedtime, yet the next morning the cupboard's almost bare.

Everyone has a slightly different reason for becoming a Night Stalker. Although the symptoms of this overeating pattern seem funny, they're not. Because most doctors would agree that when you wake up in the middle of the night to eat, your compulsive eating problem has reached a critical level.

Pete became a Night Stalker because of business worries that woke him up; he used food as a means of lulling himself back to sleep. Laura developed the Night Stalker eating pattern for a very different reason: "I come from a large family—five kids. We weren't poor, but you really had to be quick with your eating if you wanted to get a second helping, especially of something all us kids wanted, like dessert. I was one of the younger kids, and I felt my big brothers were getting an unfair share of the pie—literally.

"So I decided to beat them all to the punch. Starting when I was around ten or eleven, I'd wake up in the middle of the night, tiptoe downstairs, and take an extra portion of whatever I wanted that was left over, before my brothers got to it.

"The trick was never to let it show that you had appropriated food for yourself in the middle of the night. You'd shave off thin slivers of pie or cake, if that's what you wanted. You'd take slices of bread from the middle of the loaf, not from the ends where a missing slice would be more noticeable. As long as you didn't make noise or cooking smells, nobody would wake up and nobody would find out."

That's all well and good when you're ten years old and the runt of the litter. But when you're a thirty-seven-year-old woman, as Laura now is, it's pretty tough to beat a decades-old eating habit. Which seems all the more silly when, like Laura, you're the mistress of your own home and refrigerator and can eat what and when you want,

"It's such a dumb habit; I wish I could stop," Laura says shamefacedly. "If my husband found out, I'd be so humiliated. But I just can't stop. It's a part of my way of life."

### The Secret Snacker ☐

Laura is not just a Night Stalker. In part, she's a Secret Snacker, too. Secret Snackers do their overeating in private. When eating in public or even when eating with their families at home, Secret Snackers barely pick at their food. Yet these people are overweight. At the least they are always struggling with an incipient weight problem—five pounds up, five pounds down.

Secret Snackers' friends frequently tell them, "I don't understand how you could possibly gain weight. I never see you eat a thing." That observation is only partially correct. The Secret Snacker eats, all right. It's just that he never eats when you can see him. Part of the reason is shame—the Secret Snacker doesn't like to be seen overeating by others; it demolishes his image of himself as a well-disciplined adult, in complete control of his eating habits and of his life.

However, the crucial factor that defines the Secret Snacker eating personality is that the Secret Snacker doesn't have an excessive appetite *in public*. Those are the key words: in public. The presence of other people serves as a dramatic damper on the Secret Snacker's food consumption; in public, he eats at a normal or below-normal level. Secret Snackers can only enjoy eating—rather, enjoy overeating—when they're all by themselves, able to savor every morsel in absolute privacy.

Why is that? Perhaps it's the *way* in which they eat in private—licking, sucking, using fingers, dining sloppily—that gives them their particular satisfaction. Perhaps their Secret Snacking has elements of the Rebel personality type in it; the Secret Snacker may feel he's getting back at well-meaning friends and family who tell him not to overeat. By becoming a Secret Snacker, then, he can indulge himself in the privacy of his own psyche.

Secret Snackers are a lot like "respectable" alcoholics when it comes to the creative methods they employ in hiding their addiction. Alcoholics may develop many clever methods of hiding their liquor bottles from family and neighbors. Similarly, chronic Secret Snackers concoct elaborate schemes for hiding their sin-foods.

"I used to hide candy bars in an empty detergent box next to my dishwasher," recalls Fay, who is a chronic Secret Snacker. "I had hiding places for all these foods I wasn't supposed to eat, so my husband and kids never knew I was eating like a pig. I used to hide Vienna finger cookies inside my jewelry box, in the secret compartment. Most women would have put their diamonds or their pearls there. It all depends on what you consider valuable, I guess. To me, the cookies and the candy bars were beyond valuable. They were necessary to maintain my sanity.

"I was convinced that I had to have a backup system of candy bars or cookies or baked goods for myself—reserved exclusively for my use. I might 'need' those binge foods. And if those binge foods weren't there, I feared I might actually go crazy—climb the walls, because I ran out of Mars bars. I'm serious."

Fay turned red as she recounted how she once, in the throes of her food addiction, hid an entire Bavarian cream torte in the bottom of her clothes hamper: "I snuck away to eat it, bite by bite, while the kids were outside playing. They could never understand why Mommy always locked the screen door to the backyard, so that they couldn't just walk into the house when they wanted to get a drink or come in from playing. I locked them out, so that my children wouldn't catch me while I was ramming candy bars or cookies or cake or ice cream down my throat. If that isn't food addiction, I don't know what is."

Fay isn't alone in the Secret Snacker personality pattern, if that's any comfort to her. Secret Snackers abound—you can find them on nearly every well-manicured suburban block, in nearly every high-rise apartment building. Like Fay, other Secret Snackers are so afraid to give themselves and their guilty secret overeating away that they won't even throw the incriminating evidence into their own garbage pails for the neighbors and the garbagemen to see. All those bakery boxes, those candy wrappers, those frozen-food packages would leave tell-tale clues of overconsumption and general, all-around gluttony.

So in the dead of night, a Secret Snacker will tiptoe down his apartment building's corridors to deposit—unseen by anyone else—his guilty leavings in the incinerator. Burned up, there's no evidence of his eating transgressions. Or under cover of walking the dog or taking a leisurely stroll, a dedicated Secret Snacker will stealthily drop his ice-cream cartons and bakery boxes into the neighbors' trash cans. "Let them look guilty; let me eat cake," seems to be the Secret Snacker's slogan.

### The Junk Food Junkie ☐

This is one of the most common types of overeating personalities. Every American has been or will be a Junk Food Junkie at some point in his life. Junk food—with its highly sugared or highly salted and largely empty calories—is a seductive kind of eating experience. With every tooth-rotting and stomach-ravaging mouthful, junk food reasserts its spellbinding power over our appetites.

One reason junk foods seem so wildly attractive to us is

their illicit quality. You *know* this stuff is bad for you—it'll rot your teeth, give you pimples, or has a thousand calories to the ounce. These all-too-obvious drawbacks give junk foods a kind of subliminal mystique. You're playing with fire, as you gorge on chocolate-chip cookies and potato chips, washed down by an all-American sweet cola.

Junk foods are also highly advertised on television and other media. This increases their desirability. Television advertising aimed at children, in particular, is chock full of commercials for highly sugared cereals, candies, and other empty-calorie foods. These junk-food eating habits are thus instilled in childhood, making them doubly hard to resist in later life.

All the quintessentially American junk foods like Twinkies, potato chips, Coke, Pepsi, Fritos, and candy bars hold a cornucopia of emotional messages. Messages like: "Remember how you always used to eat Twinkies while you were watching Saturday morning TV as a little kid? Times were good then. Twinkies made those times good. Ergo, stuff those Twinkies into your face, even though you're thirty-five years old now, and you've got a spare tire around your middle big enough to fit a Mack truck."

Junk foods also carry many conformity messages and pressures within all that cellophane packaging. If "everybody else" is munching on corn chips and cola, it's pretty hard to resist conforming and sharing the junk food, in order to be "one of the guys." And all the while, every Junk Food Junkie carries in the back of his head the knowledge that these foods are nutritionally disastrous, full of empty calories, excessive sugar, salt, preservatives, artificial colorings, artificial everything.

Junk Food Junkies, though, can't really help themselves. They know junk food is bad for them, but they continue to eat it. It's quite similar to the way smokers continue to light up cigarettes, despite the warnings printed on each pack: "The Surgeon General has determined that cigarette smoking is dangerous to your health." That doesn't stop confirmed smokers. And knowledge about all the ghastly consequences of living on junk food doesn't stop true Junk Food Junkies either. If nothing else, you have to applaud their bravery.

Junk Food Junkie-hood has become a part of the national consciousness. It's no longer an in-joke; it's a social trend. There was even a hit record entitled "Junk Food Junkie," which wryly capitalized on this national bent for self-destruction via empty calories: "I pull out some Fritos, Dr. Pepper, and an old Moon Pie / And I sit back in glorious expectation of a genuine junk-food high. . . ."

A subcategory of the Junk Food Junkie personality actually does associate eating with getting high. This behavior pattern might as well be called by its slang name—the Munchies. It was dubbed this by the sixties drug culture to denote the rapacious desire for food—particularly junk foods and sweets—that often occurs after you've gotten high on marijuana. People afflicted with the Munchies, however, aren't dyed-in-the-wool overeaters. They'd probably be happier lighting up than chewing up. So they're overeaters merely by a chemical side effect of getting high, not by personality pattern.

### Lonelyhearts ☐

Loneliness is a chronic twentieth-century problem. People are lonely because of divorce and death, because of urban anonymity and suburban passivity, because the emphasis in the "Me Generation" has been on *me*, not *us*. When getting friends seems impossible and getting lovers seems improbable, many people become desperate to find a substitute for the dearth of human companionship, something tangible to fill the void. For many lonely people, it boils down to a simple equation: you can't buy your friends, but you can buy your food.

People acting out the Lonelyhearts overeating pattern substitute food for friendships. They substitute an ice-cream cone for a conversation, a hamburger for a hug, a rice pudding for a relationship, and a chocolate kiss for a flesh-and-blood kiss. By eating, the Lonelyhearts person can temporarily block out his feelings of loneliness, emptiness, and friendlessness. He's too busy swallowing, chewing, and preparing the next tidbit to think much about the fact that his telephone never rings, that he doesn't get invitations, that the only person who really loves him is his grocer— "What a nice, fat bill you've rung up, sir."

Functioning as a Lonelyhearts overeater can serve as a kind of temporary emotional anesthesia, but it can lead to a genuine inability to form real relationships. It's so much easier to deal with a slab of Camembert and some crackers than it is to deal with a real human being. And that's why some Lonelyhearts actually begin to avoid living relationships; it's so much simpler to be emotionally sustained by several thousand calories a day. Calories, after all, don't talk back, don't tell you that you're immature, and certainly don't tell you that they're leaving you for somebody who's more exciting. Thus, you can see how the Lonelyhearts lifestyle is both a comfort and a copout.

Grace became a Lonelyhearts overeater after she moved to a new city to pursue her career. All her old friends and family were back east, so at first Grace felt quite alone—and lonesome. Just when she was beginning to settle into the new city and her new job, Grace caught pneumonia. The disease put her out of social circulation for many weeks; she just didn't feel strong enough to run around after a taxing day at work. By the time Grace was fully recuperated from her pneumonia, she realized that she had lived in the new city for six months and had no good, close friends.

Grace felt despondent; she concluded that she'd never make friends in this town. She would come home each night after work and eat her way through a bag of groceries. On Saturday nights, instead of going out to meet new people, Grace would sit at home, stuffing her mouth until midnight, when she fell into bed with a carbohydrate-induced sleepiness.

Without realizing what was happening to her, Grace became a confirmed Lonelyhearts overeater. The substitution of food for friends became somewhat self-destructive for her.

Now it seemed to Grace that making the effort to get out of her apartment to make new friends was too risky, too expensive, too tiring, too time-consuming. Besides, she didn't look too good anymore—all that weight she'd put on deflated her self-confidence even further. "Who wants to be a friend to a tub of lard?" Grace asked herself before downing another cup of coffee accompanied by a thick slice of strawberry cream pie. She had come to the conclusion that "a girl's best friend is her Mallomars."

Divorce and widowing can thrust many vulnerable people into the Lonelyhearts syndrome. The concept of vulnerability is important here. People don't become Lonelyhearts because they are strong and self-confident; they turn into Lonelyhearts because they are vulnerable and, probably, oversensitive to both their feelings of loneliness and their fantasies of possible rejection if they did try to make friends.

Along with his final divorce papers, Lee got his passport into the world of the Lonelyhearts overeater. Newly divorced, Lee sits at home night after night. He's hurt because his ex-wife left him. "That must show there's something terribly wrong with me," he thinks. "Something I'm not aware of or in control of makes women think I'm a horrible person. I wish I could hide." And Lee does hide. He sits at home alone night after night, feeling thoroughly miserable about himself, wallowing in his loneliness. He idly considers going out to a bar, "but I'm out of practice at the singles scene. I wouldn't know how to behave. Besides, picking up girls always made me so nervous. I'm nervous enough without adding to my problems."

One night, Lee decides that instead of sitting home by himself, he'll get some company. He orders a pizza—large, plenty of anchovies. Eating the pizza made him feel bloated and, curiously, better, so the next night Lee orders in Chinese food and tops off this feast with some brownies. He feels better yet, much less lonely, much less pained. He has almost stopped thinking about his ex-wife.

Overeating when he's home alone at night becomes a way of life for Lee, the Lonelyhearts way of life. Food becomes his crutch and his companion. Food becomes his personal anesthesia, deadening the pain of his aloneness and loneliness. He's like a living incarnation of the "Peanuts" cartoon strip, in which a heartbroken Snoopy tries to eat his way into forgetfulness after his beagle girl friend jilts him. As Snoopy concluded: "You try for a little happiness and what do you get? A few memories and a fat stomach."

The Lonelyhearts overeaters completely reverse the old adage for weight loss of "Reach for your mate, instead of your plate." On the contrary, the Lonelyhearts eater would much rather reach for a plate, instead of a mate, pass the mashed potatoes, please. The Lonelyhearts reasoning is persuasive. After all, how many friends could you stockpile in your freezer and then heat up precisely when you *need* them? Human beings are so much less predictable, less reliable, less loyal than the ever-ready, ever-comforting foods the Lonelyhearts can buy. As the Lonelyhearts think between bites, "Who says money can't buy you love? Money *can* buy you love—if you're willing to settle for heartburn as a side effect."

### The Bargain Hunter □

This is almost a comic-relief type of overeating personality. These people aren't neurotic about food—they're driven to find bargains. These are people who clip coupons, who watch the newspaper for weekly specials at the supermarket, butcher shop, and bake shop, who can't pass by food if the sign on the shelf says "reduced." That's how the Bargain Hunter overeater ends up eating things he never dreamed of and in quantities he never dreamed of—just to take advantage of a bargain. Calorically speaking, their food bargains take advantage of them!

Neal isn't supposed to eat fried foods, not after his last gall-bladder attack. But Neal sees an ad in the paper—one dollar off on every family-pack order at Kentucky Fried Chicken. So Neal trots in and buys a "bargain" family pack. It doesn't occur to him at this point that (a) he doesn't have a family to eat it with him and (b) his gall bladder hates fried stuff. Nevertheless, Neal eats all the bargain-priced gall-bladder no-nos like mashed potatoes with thick gravy and coleslaw with mayonnaise, not to mention the famed finger-lickin' fried chicken. Neal never could resist a bargain—a dollar off!

Somehow, it seems like less of a money-saving proposition to Neal after he has had a gall-bladder attack, had to spend $50 on a doctor's visit, and had to shell out about $20 on new and expensive medication to ease the pain. Some bargains cost a lot more than you think at first bite.

Another chronic Bargain Hunter is Mitzi. She's on a diet of sorts—she's *always* on a diet . . . of sorts. Mitzi is trying to cut down on her calories, even though she eats many of her meals out. One day she spots two coupons in her local paper; the coupons proclaim a real bargain: order one burger and fries at Burger King, and you get a free burger. Never one to pass up a bargain, Mitzi redeems one of the two coupons. She just can't restrain her bargain-hunting soul, diet or no diet. So Mitzi winds up eating an order of fries and *two* Whopper Juniors with cheese. After all, one of those Whopper Juniors with cheese is free—free!

"Well, it could have been worse, calorically speaking." Mitzi smiles. "The other coupon in the paper was for two Whoppers plus fries. I figured by limiting myself to the coupon for two Whopper *Juniors,* I was practicing moderation—and still getting a great bargain. Boy, do my jeans feel snug. I wonder why. . . ."

That's the last of our overeating personality types. If you've been keeping score of how closely you resemble each eating type, you can now compile your own personal overeating profile. Go back and look at the numbers you've recorded in the box next to each eating personality type. The higher you've scored yourself on a personality, the more you resemble that overeating type.

Take the five scores in which you judged yourself closest to a specific type—your five highest scores on the ten-point scale. Write down which overeating types those are, in descending order of your score.

Now you've got, right before you, the principal dimensions of your *own* overeating patterns. This combination comprises your own distinctive overeating personality type.

Now that you know your own overeating syndromes, you can recognize when you're heading toward overeating. But now you're not defenseless against the onslaught of overeating desires. You're alert, you're aware—and you're prepared to help yourself.

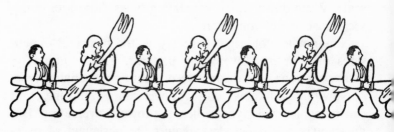

# 9 Eating Personalities: The Undereaters

It takes two hefty chapters to cover overeating personalities. But undereaters occupy only one rather slim chapter. It's not just that heavier people—the overeaters—take up more room, but that there are more of them. Undereaters are a minority group. In fact, people with classic "good eating habits" are probably the smallest minority group of any eating personality category.

Most of us have a vague idea of good eating habits and proper nutrition. We may waffle a bit on the subject: "Doesn't that have something to do with getting green and yellow vegetables, citrus fruits, protein, and a glass of milk every day?" But very few people actually practice good eating habits and good nutrition consistently. Not even dietitians do. (And this isn't meant to cast aspersions on dietitians, but as a group this profession, too, seems to have a disproportionate number of overweight members.)

Just because a person has an undereating personality type, it doesn't mean that he or she eats properly balanced meals. Undereaters can be just as malnourished as overeaters who gorge on the "empty" calories of junk foods and snacks. And not all undereaters are skinny—not by a long shot. Very, very few people are consistent undereaters. The most dramatic example of perpetual undereaters are those who suffer from the psychological disorder known as anorexia nervosa, but more about that later. Most people who display undereating syndromes are only part-time undereaters. The rest of the time, they're either eating normal, fairly well-balanced meals. Or they're stuffing their faces, just like the rest of us. Most overeaters succumb to undereating syndromes at certain points in their lives. These are the times when "the weight just seemed to roll off" without resorting to conscious dieting.

## The Ramadan Faster ▢

Ramadan is the Islamic religion's yearly month-long period of fasting. During Ramadan, no good Moslem will eat—during the daylight hours. But the minute the sun goes down, all calories break loose. The faithful who have fasted all day long shovel special Ramadan delicacies into their mouths until late at night.

You don't have to follow Islam to be a Ramadan Faster. In Western cultures, the Ramadan Faster just can't find time to eat during the daytime. But once he settles down at home in the evening, the feast goes on nonstop.

Sheila is a Ramadan Faster type of undereater. She teaches third grade at an understaffed inner-city school. Usually, Sheila wakes up too late to get any breakfast before she bounds off to work. During the day she abstains from eating, too. She hates dining in the teachers' lounge: "By that time, my sandwich is soggy and lukewarm, and I really don't like sandwiches all that much to begin with. I'd rather eat a green salad or an omelette for lunch. So long as I don't *like* what I have to eat at lunch, I decided it was better not to eat then at all." So lunch hour passes for Sheila with a couple cups of coffee—"black with two packets of Sweet 'n' Low in each."

During the afternoons, Sheila teaches her class on a completely empty stomach. But that doesn't bother her. "Oh, sure, at first I used to be *ravenous* by the time three o'clock rolled around. But after a semester or so, I got used to not eating. I never notice getting hungry anymore. Well, sometimes my stomach does start making these growling noises. That's really embarrassing when you're teaching forty hyperactive eight-year-olds. But I don't associate that growling with hunger anymore. It's just a funny noise that my stomach sometimes makes."

When she gets home, Sheila fixes dinner for her husband and daughter. And then Sheila really tucks it in: "I eat anything that's not nailed down: a couple of rolls with butter, a huge salad, meat, dessert. It's almost a shock to the system to get all that food pouring in when you've shrunk your stomach the whole day long. But that feeling doesn't stop me from eating."

Sheila follows the Ramadan Faster undereating pattern all through the school year. Yet she's not particularly slender. She wears a size 12, but considering how often Sheila abstains from eating, you'd expect her to be a marvelously bony size 6. Where then does the flesh on Sheila's bones come from? Sheila answers with an embarrassed smile: "I can't stop eating during the school vacations. Without having my day occupied by teaching, I just cook and nibble and eat everything I shouldn't. Summer is the worst time. I have a real thing for ice cream. All brands, all flavors, just so long as it's ice cream." She pats her stomach. "You have no idea how many pounds ice cream alone can put on you. It's really depressing!"

### The Workaholic ☐

This undereating personality type often behaves very much like the Ramadan Faster. The Workaholic is so busy with work—whether it's housework, child-rearing, sales calls, or conferences—that he or she literally *forgets* to eat. Sometimes this Workaholic undereating pattern can last for years—until the undereater switches to a less demanding job or life-style. Or the Workaholic undereating pattern can persist only during the "busy season" of the undereater's business.

Marianne slipped into the Workaholic undereating syndrome quite accidentally when she received a much-sought-after promotion to a programming executive position in a national broadcasting chain. Broadcasting is a so-called glamor industry, so the competition for jobs within it is fierce. It's also a field that has traditionally excluded women from decision-making positions in programming. So Marianne was both flattered and terrified when she received her promotion. Flattered that she had broken through the industry's barriers to women and terrified that she would fail and be fired. For broadcasting is glamorous but job security is notoriously fragile, with executives being replaced as in a game of musical chairs.

Marianne was determined to succeed, so she took to spending long hours at her office. She arrived early and breakfasted on a quick cup of coffee and a few bites of a doughnut. She was literally so involved in her work that she didn't notice that the doughnut lay half-eaten on her desk.

Lunch often consisted of business meetings—expense-account opulence at fashionable restaurants. But Marianne still didn't end up eating very much: "I was so busy trying to score points at lunch meetings that I really couldn't have cared less what food was put before me. I was too busy psyching out colleagues or the competition to care about how succulent the steak was or if the soufflé was divine. And once my adrenaline started revving up during lunch, whatever appetite I had just vanished."

Marianne worked late most nights. If she remembered, she sent out for a sandwich before the nearby delis closed for the evening. More often than not, Marianne forgot to order anything at all for dinner: "So either I would just skip dinner, or I'd get something gruesome-tasting from the vending machines in the hall."

By the time she dragged herself back to her apartment, Marianne was too exhausted to consider cooking. Sometimes she'd stop by a late-night sandwich shop and pick up a light meal. Other times she'd just satisfy her hunger with an apple and a small piece of cheese that languished in her almost-empty refrigerator.

Marianne maintained this unconscious undereating pattern even on those frequent occasions when she'd have to attend a business-related cocktail party or reception: "It was the same deal as at lunch. I was too busy trying to keep on top of things to really tuck into hors d'oeuvres and such. During the whole time I had that job, food pretty much lost its meaning for me. I was so completely absorbed in my work that I really didn't have *time* to fantasize about all the great food I was missing. My work was so satisfying—and so overwhelming—that I very seldom ever felt a real need to eat."

Marianne didn't even notice she'd lost weight from her Workaholic patterns until she went home for Christmas and her newly skinny frame was cause for concern and clucking in her family. "After I returned to my job, I tried to eat properly, but my good intentions lasted about a week." She lapsed into the Workaholic syndrome again without really noticing it.

For over two years, Marianne kept on eating—rather, not eating—in this fashion. At that point, she changed jobs, changed companies, and soon found she was getting paid more but actually had less work to do. Now that she felt relatively seasoned as a broadcasting programming executive, Marianne began to notice that she could order great meals on her expense account. She started eating, even becoming something of a gourmet regarding Japanese and Far Eastern cuisines.

Not surprisingly, Marianne gained back some of the weight she had shed while living the Workaholic undereating syndrome. The ultrasvelte figure she had learned to take for granted began to acquire some unwanted adipose padding. Not very much, but eight pounds or so. Enough to make Marianne feel stuffed into her clothes. Only then did she sit down and analyze how she had changed her life-style and her eating habits when she changed jobs. And only then did Marianne pinpoint the source of her enviably slender figure.

Ray is a seasonal Workaholic undereater. He is a partner in a smallish dress-manufacturing firm. In the "rag trade," seasonal business highs are the rule. During the busy seasons for his firm when the new summer and fall lines come out, Ray forgets about food, forgets about eating, even forgets about strawberry milk shakes (his favorite nosh). "All I can think about then is getting the new line ready to show. And after that, I think about convincing the buyers that they should buy our dresses for their stores, instead of somebody else's."

Ray and his partners work themselves into a frenzy during their busy seasons. Their offices and showroom are excitingly chaotic for weeks on end. "We work such long hours then, that I couldn't care less whether I ate a big dinner or a big lunch or not. I've got more important things to think about. Like whether or not we're going to go into bankruptcy if some department store chain cancels its order. When business gets that thrilling, who needs food?"

During the rest of the year, Ray eats and overeats just like the typical American. But during the busy seasons, he's a genuine Workaholic undereater. Ray veers between (relative) feast and (actual) famine in his seasonal eating patterns. As the year's caloric surpluses balance out the year's caloric deficiencies, Ray is able to keep stylishly trim; he wears the same size suit as he did when he was married almost twenty years ago. "My only real trouble," Ray jokes, "is where do you find a ready-made, good-fitting suit in a 37 short?"

## Romeo and Juliet □

The most pleasant form of undereating behavior occurs in people who are joyously "suffering" from the Romeo and Juliet personality pattern. These undereaters are, literally, love-starved. In this case, love-starved doesn't mean a lack of love. No, with the Romeo and Juliet personality, love-starved means that the lover has simply lost his or her appetite because of sheer passion. For most people, falling in love is apparently even better than Dexedrine for cutting the appetite in half.

157

Almost everyone has experienced the Romeo and Juliet variety of undereating at some brief period in his life. Remember when you first fell in love? Besides the feeling of euphoria, the semidelirious feelings of well-being, there are other distinct, measurable symptoms of falling in love. Among them are sweaty palms, a pounding heart, and increased pulse rate when you see your beloved. Another recognizable symptom is loss of appetite. Desire for the loved one cancels out the desire for food. As the old song goes, "You're not sick; you're just in love."

When people first fall in love, they tend to be so wrapped up in each other—in thought as well as in body—that the craving to eat (and overeat) ebbs away. Recall how you and your new lover planned a superromantic, candlelit dinner for two at an intimate French restaurant. And then you both virtually forgot to eat the food as you gazed passionately into each other's love-glazed eyes, as you held hands across the table. Maybe those suffering from the Romeo and Juliet undereating syndrome can force themselves to sip at a glass of wine over dinner together—the better to loosen up the libido. But consume a large meal? Hardly.

Clearly, then, when you've first fallen in love, the taste of the beloved's lips perks you up far more than the taste of a four-course French meal, no matter how expertly prepared. Maybe that results in another reason new lovers feel so good physically. As if by magic they shed excess pounds and become trimmer and fitter. At least temporarily, at least until the glow of love fades.

### The Worry Wart ☐

Just as love can cause loss of appetite, other emotions can also induce undereating behavior. The Worry Wart personality undereaters literally worry their lips and stomachs shut. Tension, anxiety, depression—emotional black clouds in general—can cause even a confirmed overeater to skip meals, even to stop eating altogether.

Cheryl is a classic Worry Wart undereater. As her emotional tension and depression rise, her appetite declines. It's a direct inverse relationship. "After my husband and I have a fight or if one of the kids gets into trouble at school, I get so nervous, I can just feel a huge lump rising up in my throat. It's as if that lump blocks off my appetite and all my desire to eat. I don't quite feel sick to my stomach, but I can get so nervous that even if I *force* myself to eat, everything tastes like unsalted cardboard cartons—disgusting. I get nervous an awful lot lately. My marriage is in trouble, and I have two teenagers who are getting kind of wild. Both those things combined would make anybody lose their appetite, don't you think?"

Cheryl is the envy of her friends, because she never has to diet in order to maintain her trim shape. "All my girl friends ask for my diet secret," Cheryl sighs. "But how can I tell them that I don't do it with willpower—I do it with worry?"

Not everyone displays such omnipresent Worry Wart undereating behavior as Cheryl, but most of us have experienced this syndrome at moments of intense stress. For instance, when a loved one is in a hospital undergoing an operation, few people want to leave the waiting room and go down to the hospital cafeteria for a snack or meal. And they probably wouldn't want to go even if hospital food *were* edible.

Or consider the situation of high-school seniors, sweating out the weeks of agonizing tension before receiving college acceptance or rejection. This degree of anxiety is quite enough to send even normally ravenous teenagers into the Worry Wart undereating life-style.

Worry, tension, and anxiety serve to dry up the taste buds. Sure, you can taste the food, but higher emotional needs have superseded most of the emotional impulses to eat. A slighter degree of anxiety or tension would cause most chronic overeaters to run for the refrigerator, but great emotional stress has a damper effect, blunting the desire to eat.

# The Shrinking Violet ☐

"I just can't get anything to stay down" is the line the Shrinking Violet repeats most often to family, friends, lovers, and anybody else who will listen and give sympathy. This type of undereater associates lack of appetite and underweight with getting love and attention. His thinking seems to run like this: as the stomach shrinks, the lovability expands.

Kelly is an archetypal Shrinking Violet. As the fourth of five children, she often felt, as a child, that she didn't get much attention from her parents. "I wasn't the baby of the family, but I wasn't one of the big kids either, so I felt pretty much left out and ignored," she recalls. As a small child, Kelly was naturally slender and delicate in appearance. But this physical delicacy became a cause for her parents' genuine concern when Kelly came down with pneumonia. She was very ill for several weeks and came out of the pneumonia with a definite frailty, due to the weight she had lost during the course of the illness.

Her pediatrician said it was vital that Kelly gain back the weight she had lost; otherwise, her health might be seriously and permanently impaired. "So my mother made it her major concern to see that I ate more, so that I'd put some flesh back on my bones," Kelly remembers. "Mom would spend what seemed like hours sitting next to me, cajoling me into swallowing the next bite and the next. I never had so much undivided attention from my mother before, and I must admit, I grew to like it."

Very soon, the little girl learned that she could get attention and affection by claiming she had no appetite, that she couldn't possibly eat anything, that the sight of food made her nauseous. For years after she'd recovered from pneumonia, Kelly kept using her no-appetite routine to become the center of attention at family dinners. "It was the one surefire way to stand out when you're one of five kids. Sometimes I actually didn't have an appetite, and so I didn't eat. Then my mother, my father, my older sister and brothers would all try to make me eat. I have to confess that at other times, I just pretended that the thought of food made me sick to my stomach. I intentionally acted pathetic to get more attention."

Even when she grew older, Kelly kept up her Shrinking Violet act. It had become a way of life for her, this very noticeable complaining about her lack of appetite. "When I got sick at college or got real worried about final exams, I would just very conspicuously stop eating and lose weight. I'd make myself get even skinnier than I already was. And just to make sure my friends would notice, I'd make big, sighing speeches about how I wished I could get some solid food down, just a few crumbs—because I was starving to death but too nervous to eat."

These Shrinking Violet gambits worked like a charm in attracting the desired special attention for Kelly: "My roommates would always start clucking over me, trying to get me to eat, just the way my mother had. And the fellows I went out with went crazy for that routine. With them, it was always 'You poor angel, you need somebody to take care of you and see that you eat to keep your strength.' Of course, my being so fragile-looking was definitely a turn-on for most of those guys."

For Kelly, it paid to be an undereater. It paid in terms of increased attention, extra sexual desirability, and a favorable body shape. ("Slender is beautiful" is one of our society's favorite unspoken sayings.) When Kelly left college, her Shrinking Violet personality pattern paid off monetarily, too. Reed-slim with an excellent (and prominent) bone structure, Kelly shifted rather easily into the lucrative career of a high-fashion model. She earns $100 an hour, posing for photographers. Kelly has won the biggest possible payoff for a Shrinking Violet, using her skinniness and tiny appetite to make herself special, envied, loved, and even to achieve minor celebrityhood.

While the Shrinking Violet can turn her appetite on and off pretty much at will, the persons with the next undereating behavior pattern aren't in such self-control and aren't as lucky. Not by a long shot.

## The Distorted Mirror: Anorexia Nervosa ☐

The other undereating personality types we've discussed in this chapter have all been within fairly normal to mildly neurotic emotional ranges. However, anorexia nervosa is a far more serious, potentially life-threatening psychophysiological disease. Anorexia nervosa has received numerous diagnoses, and physicians are not in complete agreement on the causes of the condition. But it does primarily affect young upper-middle-class and upper-class women, aged eleven to twenty-four.

At first, the potential anorexic (as those with this condition are called) seems just an unusually zealous dieter. But the anorexic is caught up in the Pursuit of Thin far more than an emotionally healthy young woman would be. The anorexic has a distorted perception of her own body. Even when she goes below eighty pounds, as many anorexics do, the sufferer will look at herself in the mirror and think she's of normal weight or even pudgy. She psychologically disregards the mirror's physical evidence: that she has acquired a concentration-camp boniness, pallor, and weakness. She has become grotesquely emaciated, ready to die for the sake of being "slim enough."

Anorexia nervosa goes far beyond mere dieting carried to an absurd extent. The anorexic does not really lose her appetite. Instead, she becomes obsessed with food, and, therefore, obsessed with avoiding it. Doctors say that anorexics dream about food, feel hunger, and are often pathologically obsessed with their food consumption—or the lack thereof.

"Starvation is merely a symptom and not the real problem," cautions Dr. Hilde Bruch, an authority on eating disorders who is a professor of psychiatry at the Baylor University College of Medicine. "The real illness has to do with how you feel about yourself. There are many underlying personality conflicts."

Many psychiatrists believe that anorexics undereat so severely because they want to avoid growing up. Anorexia nervosa accomplishes this bizarre wish on several levels.

Since the typical anorexic is afraid of participating in adult sexuality, she diets so strenuously that her body loses all womanly curves. Her breasts literally shrivel up (most mammary tissue is fat anyway). And eventually amenorrhea (total cessation of menstruation) occurs. The anorexic has transformed herself from a blooming adolescent or young woman into a mock-child: flat-chested, weak, gangly, asexual.

The anorexic's willful starvation of herself makes her a child again in other, more subtle ways. Most anorexics feel they are unable to cope with the world as fully participating adults. They would like to remain dependent upon their parents, yet at the same time often harbor a secret wish to punish them.

Through anorexia nervosa, the victim of the Distorted Mirror syndrome can have it both ways. She can have her cake and never eat it, too. This is achieved because physically the anorexic becomes a helpless, waiflike creature. Everybody is ready to pay attention to her: "How weak you look, darling" or "Please, try to eat something for Mother's sake, dear." She becomes the object of solicitude, fit only to be pitied and cared for.

At times, some anorexics say they can feel the logical part of their personality wanting to eat, wanting to get well. Yet they also experience another, irrational facet of the personality forbidding the consumption of food, forbidding healthful weight gain, forbidding cure. The possible existence of logical/healthful impulses opposing a suicidal/self-punishing personality aspect has led some psychiatrists to say that anorexia nervosa is nothing more than schizophrenia for rich, skinny girls. Anorexics have been treated by a variety of methods, including behavior modification, psychotherapy, and hospitalization for intravenous feeding to sustain life.

The real sickness and tragedy of anorexia nervosa comes through most clearly when you talk to an anorexic. Patrice has been anorexic for seven years. Her symptoms of self-starvation began when she was seventeen: "I had just fallen in love for the first time, and I was all open and vulnerable, the way you can be only the first time. Well, the boy hurt me really badly. He hurt me so badly that I decided I would never let anyone hurt me that way again."

Patrice's solution to her broken love affair: falling into the Distorted Mirror personality pattern. "I was 5 foot 6 and 128 pounds then. I thought I was grossly overweight. So little by little, I dieted down to where I am now—76 pounds. No, I don't feel very skinny. In fact, when I look at myself, I feel I look perfectly normal or maybe even slightly overweight."

Patrice is not a stupid young woman. She got good grades at college, until her extreme underweight made her too weak to attend classes. "I couldn't walk across campus anymore. I couldn't walk up steps to get to lectures, and once I got there, I was too weak to take notes or study. I also was worried about being exposed to so many people. The doctors told me I was so underweight and malnourished that if I even caught a cold, I'd have no resistance. It'd turn into pneumonia, and I'd die. And I may be many things, but I'm not suicidal, not really."

That statement is hard to accept when Patrice relates her bizarre undereating life-style: "I keep a detailed log in which I write down every single calorie that I've consumed all day. I weigh and measure my food with little scales like they use at Weight Watchers. I don't allow myself any meat or starches. The closest I come to carbohydrates is an apple or orange every day and some measured portions of dietetic gelatin. Each serving of that is one and a half calories, but you have to watch it, because those calories add up. I allow myself to eat *exactly* 776⅓ calories every day. No more. That way I won't gain weight. It's precisely enough to keep me at 76 pounds."

Even with this severely restricted caloric intake, Patrice uses other self-punishing devices to maintain her weight. She is a secret vomiter. "No, not really a secret vomiter. I don't hide it." She notes with a strange pride, "I have learned over the years to vomit at will. I won't keep down any food unless I want to, even if the doctors force it down my throat. I'm happy at my present weight."

The only trouble with Patrice's "happiness" is that her doctors say she is on the verge of death. When such severe underweight is sustained for long periods, the body consumes its own fat tissues first. When the fat is completely depleted, the body, in its desperate search for fuel, begins to feed upon itself. Muscle-wasting results; the anorexic "eats" her own muscles to survive.

The trouble is that when muscular organs like the heart are "eaten," death cannot be far behind. This happened in 1978 to a New Jersey anorexic. She had starved herself from 120 pounds down to 69 pounds. Her body consumed parts of her heart muscle. The anorexic suffered a heart attack as a result, then lapsed into coma. She experienced another heart attack while in coma and died. The anorexic was fourteen years old.

The Distorted Mirror is undoubtedly the most severe and harmful form of undereating. If you recognize this personality type in yourself or in a friend or relative, get medical assistance immediately. Anorexia nervosa is a difficult condition to treat and may require medical supervision for many years until the anorexic has completely recovered and relearned how to eat for health.

"In a sense, a recovered anorexic is a lot like a recovered alcoholic," says one former anorexic who is now herself a physician. "The recovered alcoholic always lives with the specter of falling off the wagon and hitting the bottle again. The recovered anorexic is always afraid she'll look in the mirror and see herself as fat and ugly. And then she won't have any control again. She'll starve herself to death and be unable to stop herself. Not even to save her own life."

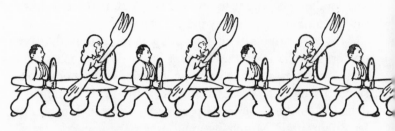

# 10  Sabotage: The Secret Ways Emotions Make Us Eat

Worrying about your weight problem is common. Solving your weight problem permanently is highly *un*common. Fewer than 10 percent of the people who lose ten pounds or more on a diet can proudly proclaim two years later that they've kept those pounds off. And almost everyone knows how difficult, how exasperating, how downright torturous it often is to stay on a diet day after day, week after week.

Why is it so very hard to change our patterns of overeating, our cycle of feast and famine, diet and binge? One significant reason is that most people are very successful, not at dieting, but at sabotaging themselves. Consciously—but more often unconsciously—most people engage in a self-defeating series of alibis, rationalizations, and tricks on themselves. These are the same people who say, "I want to lose weight and keep it off. I really do." But their unconscious drives still propel these people toward fathood, not away from it.

Why then is the classic compulsive eating pattern so resistant to change? Why do people sabotage their own weight-loss efforts? Because most people are afraid of changing themselves and of having to alter their self-image in the process. Because most people are threatened by the idea of changing their whole way of eating—and hence their whole way of living—so they develop these self-sabotage tricks to defeat themselves.

One reason many people repeatedly regain lost weight or break their diets is that they're subsconsciously afraid of getting thin. Just as there's such a thing as fear of success, there's such a thing as fear of thinness. Fear of thinness arises from the anxiety about the unknown changes that may be in store for us if we change our physical shape to conform more closely to this society's ideal—the thin body. For some people, thinness means that they won't be able to hide behind their weight any longer. There will be no more wooden-leg excuses: "If only I were thin, I'd be popular." Or "If only I lost weight, I'd have a great sex life." Or "If only I were slimmer, I could get a better job." If people who make these excuses really did succeed in becoming thin, the consequences would be more threatening, more terrifying to them than a lifetime of overweight.

Others sabotage themselves subconsciously by fearing what their sustained weight loss will mean to their loved ones. These self-sabotagers concoct rationalizations like: "My mother will be insulted if I don't eat all her special meals—she works so hard cooking them for us." Or "My husband won't have to defend me from other people's insults about my appearance, and he'll stop caring for me." Or "My children won't listen to me if I'm not a big, commanding figure."

These self-sabotaging excuses show how being overweight has become these persons' basic role in their families and in their own lives. They may be endangering their family's equilibrium if they can no longer be labeled "the chubby one" or scapegoated as "fatso, the moral weakling."

For still other compulsive eaters, emotional overeating and breaking diets can serve as a form of subconscious masochism. What is masochistic overeating? It's destroying your hard-won slimness by gorging. These people literally eat themselves sick. They may feel they don't "deserve" the happiness of thinness. So they overeat. So they gain back the pounds they fought so hard to take off. In the more severe cases of masochistic overeating, people may use compulsive eating as a very slow, very quiet form of suicide. They eat themselves to death.

Most of us, of course, don't go *that* far in our attempts to sabotage our own weight-control programs. We resort to less drastic but still very effective tricks. We play these tricks on ourselves, because we're not 100 percent certain we *want* to get thin.

Here are some of the most common tricks that would-be thin people play on themselves to remain overweight:

**Miracle Cure.** This trick on yourself consists of looking for a magical, sure cure for overweight. The self-saboteur avidly collects every new fad-diet book, every mail-order capsule that guarantees to melt off fat, every sweat-yourself-skinny body suit. These people join health clubs and try one diet group after another. Instead of putting their (considerable) efforts into solving the problems that make them overeat, they keep searching, in vain, for somebody else's miracle cure. But there are no miracle cures for obesity, not even at Lourdes.

**All or Nothing at All.** In this self-sabotaging trick, the dieter falls off the path of virtue (i.e., starvation) and then figures, "What the heck. As long as I've sinned, I may as well sin big." So if they break their diet by eating one doughnut, they figure they might as well eat the other five doughnuts in the box. This type of self-saboteur also figures if he goes off the diet at any time during the day, he might as well overeat until the next morning. So if he has a nondiet breakfast, say pancakes with maple syrup, he'll have pie for lunch and hollandaise sauce at dinner, because "I've already blown my diet for today."

**The Exercise Trick.** In this self-sabotage technique, the person tells himself it's all right to eat something forbidden on his diet, because "I'll exercise off those calories." He figures, "I'll exercise off that candy bar." Or he figures, "I'm going to start jogging tomorrow, so I can eat more and still not gain weight."

The trouble with this rationalization is that it takes an awful lot of exercise to work off even a standard 1½-ounce Hershey bar, which has about 185 calories. A 165-pound man has to walk three miles to work off one crummy chocolate bar. That's where the "perfect logic" of the Exercise Trick descends into self-sabotage. Nobody could possibly exercise enough to keep all those binge calories from taking up residence on their thighs, hips, and stomach.

**The Overdose Trick.** In this form of self-sabotage, you tell yourself it's perfectly all right to overeat enormously on one particular favorite binge food. You rationalize, "I'll eat so much of this that I'll OD on chocolate mousse/cheesecake/crackers/whatever. I'll eat so much of it that I'll never want to eat it again." The Overdose Trick actually works—temporarily—for a few people. But for most people, this self-sabotage trick only serves to camouflage a plain, old-fashioned eating binge.

**The Crutch Trick.** In this self-sabotage scheme, the overweight person can't afford to get thin. Subconsciously, she uses her fat as a crutch. Being overweight absolves her from risking failure. The kind of person who plays the Crutch Trick keeps telling herself, "If only I were thin(ner), everything would be just fine."

But what if she does get thin, and she still doesn't get the rewards she thought thinness would bring? What if she gets thin(ner) and she still isn't popular or beautiful, or gets passed over for that job promotion? Then she would have to face up to her own personal inadequacies.

It's far less frightening for her to stay overweight. By having heaviness as a crutch, she doesn't have to acknowledge her personal shortcomings or the possibility of failure. The Crutch Trick is a widely popular self-sabotage ploy for many dieters.

• • •

**Instant Skinny.** This person self-sabotages himself by demanding an instantaneous change—in his appearance, in his clothing size, in the poundage his scale registers. But most diets don't result in instant weight loss. Very often losing weight is an excruciatingly slow process, frequently studded with weeks at weight plateaus where the dieter is still starving but the pounds are still sticking. The person who wants Instant Skinny becomes fatalistic if his diet doesn't work immediately or consistently. He gets discouraged and gives up the diet altogether. And thus, he's shot himself down, doomed himself to failure by giving up.

**The Super Willpower Trick.** The person using this strategy succeeds at self-sabotage by expecting unrealistic, superhuman levels of willpower. She doesn't eliminate the leftover fattening foods from her kitchen shelves when she starts on a diet. She leaves the cake mixes and the Fritos right there in plain sight—she will be strong and not indulge. She doesn't plan her diet menus ahead or take a brown-bag, low-calorie lunch to work. Instead, she eats the same meals that her family does ("I'll just have to be strong and resist eating the fattening foods") and goes to a fast-food restaurant with her co-workers ("I can diet that way—I'll just leave the bun off my Big Mac"). If she's really good at the Super Willpower Trick, she can sabotage herself by finally allowing herself special diet foods—but only the blandest, most boring, and least appetizing diet foods possible.

By setting her willpower standards unrealistically high, this person sets the seal on her own defeat. Wantpower almost invariably triumphs over willpower where food is concerned. By expecting herself to have ironclad willpower defenses, the person playing the Super Willpower Trick on herself gives herself no defenses at all. When her willpower crumbles, she quits the diet; she fails.

**Nervous Wreck.** This method of self sabotage has some basis in physiology. Suddenly cutting down on refined sugar when you're used to a lot of it can send you into depression, feelings of weakness, or excessive irritability. But the Nervous Wreck self-saboteur makes these reactions into a fine art for self-defeat. He *knows* that when he goes on a diet, he gets grouchy. He yells at his employees. He yells at his kids. He yells at his dog. He *knows* being on a diet will get him so nervous, he won't be able to sleep nights and then his efficiency at work, not to mention his golf scores, will suffer horrendously.

The Nervous Wreck doesn't just get himself nervous. He gets the people around him nervous because of his own super-sensitivity and irritability once he goes on a diet-deprivation regime.

How is this self-sabotage? His nerves will eventually snap. He'll *have* to go off the diet to save his sanity. Actually, the person playing the Nervous Wreck Trick on himself has generated even more tension than the average dieter experiences (which is pretty considerable anyway). He has subconsciously created such monumental nervousness in order to have an excuse to go off his diet.

**Tomorrow Never Comes.** These people are big on making diet plans. They carefully research the various diets, make a study of nutrition, consider the emotional hurdles to dieting. They prepare and prepare, so that their attempt at weight loss will be successful.

So how is this a self-sabotage trick? Because these people prepare for the diet, but they always promise themselves that they'll start the diet tomorrow or next week after they've finished writing that big report or after Cousin Jody's wedding. With these people, tomorrow never comes. And the day to start the diet never comes. And so the weight loss never comes either.

**The Invalid Trick.** These people defeat themselves by claiming they have a health problem that prevents them from dieting and losing weight. Perhaps they have low blood sugar. Perhaps sudden deprivation of refined sugars and starches makes them feel weak or nauseous. These are legitimate physical responses that some people feel after they begin a diet.

But the person who plays the Invalid Trick on himself sees thinness and health as mutually exclusive. Subconsciously, they see heaviness—"some meat on those bones"—as an indication of health and strength. When they've dieted enough to be able to discern ribs and hipbones jutting through the flab, people who play the Invalid Trick suddenly feel sick. They become so anxious that their new thinness will weaken their health that they convince themselves that the diet—even a sensible, well-balanced diet—is making them sick. And so they have to go off it. For the sake of their health.

You can sidestep some of these more common methods of self-sabotage just by being aware that they exist. It also helps to keep a few basic truths in mind:

1. You must accept the fact that weight loss doesn't occur consistently. You can have some weight loss one week and none the next. This is perfectly normal and natural, and so you shouldn't let it deter you from persisting until you've reached your goal weight.

2. You have to be realistic about how perfectly you—or anybody else—can stick to a diet. No one can diet "perfectly" every day. So if you have momentary lapses, accept them as proof of your human fallibility, not as proof of being weak-willed or inferior.

3. You must sit down and decide what you want to get from your eventual weight loss. Then ask yourself how realistic these expectations are. If you're expecting the sun, the moon, and the stars as your reward for losing weight, you're bound to be sorely disappointed—which can lead you to overeat some more.

Losing weight won't make you instantly popular or sexually confident or physically gorgeous. So whittle down your unrealistic expectations, and you can reduce both your waistline and your chances for falling into self-sabotage tricks.

Of course, even if you avoid the traps of self-sabotage, you still run the risk of sabotage from outside sources. Your family and friends may be uncomfortable when you decide to shed pounds. Because when you shed pounds, you'll also be shedding the role of family fatty—the person they can feel superior to just by virtue of being thinner. While you are the family fatty, your family and spouse may feel certain of your affections. Because who else will want a fatso for a lover or best friend?

But once you become thinner, you're considered more desirable to other people both as a friend and as a lover. So your spouse, family, and friends may become worried— you're no longer a sure thing, now that you have the potential choice of leaving them for someone else. These are the kinds of pressures that can cause your loved ones to consciously or unconsciously sabotage your weight-loss plans.

Some studies estimate that as many as 20 percent of all teenagers on weight-control programs have either or both their parents tempting them with forbidden, fattening foods. The fathers seem to fear that they'll be losing their "little girls" when their adolescent daughters shed weight and become shapely. Sabotaging mothers of teenage girls may subconsciously fear that their own youth and attractiveness are being threatened by a thinner, more sexually desirable daughter. Other parents may subconsciously sabotage their children in order to keep the teenagers more dependent, feeling that overweight adolescents are less likely to leave the family because they aren't acceptable to their peers.

Surprisingly, at least one University of Wisconsin Medical School study showed that husbands of women who lost large amounts of weight were *not* happy because of their wives' new slimness. Rather, the women's large weight loss caused their husbands to be so upset that many couples divorced or separated, and other pairs suffered from problems ranging from infidelity to jealousy to impotence. As the wives became more attractive by losing weight, their husbands began to be afraid that their wives would leave them or make new demands (whether financial, social, or sexual). Many of these husbands resorted to sabotage techniques. Not because they hated their wives, but because they wanted to *keep* them, and felt too insecure or inferior to keep a slim spouse.

Thus, you can see that when spouses or families sabotage your diet, they don't do it out of hate. On the contrary, they do it largely out of misguided love.

Here are some of the most common sabotage techniques used by your family and friends. Be aware of them. And be forewarned!

**Contradictory Messages.** This is a kind of sabotage by ambivalence. Your spouse or parent tells you repeatedly, "You'd look so fantastic if only you could knock off those extra pounds." But at the same time, they keep stocking the pantry with pastries and the freezer with ice cream (your favorite flavor, too). This presence of constant temptation makes dieting difficult, if not impossible. A variation of the Contradictory Messages sabotage finds your family or spouse praising your successful dieting efforts. But then they reward you with a gift of candy or a big, fattening celebration dinner. All to commemorate your (very) temporary weight loss.

**Policeman.** This kind of saboteur nags you so much to keep on your diet—monitoring your food intake, scolding you for your lapses—that you may go off your **diet** in sheer rebellion. Just to prove that you have control over your own food intake. But you don't have control, not even when you binge—because it's still the Policeman saboteur who's controlling you.

**Homebody.** This type of saboteur tries to keep the dieter in the stifling role of Homebody, a role that will defeat the family fatty's diet plans. In the Homebody sabotage, your spouse or parents may discourage you from attending diet group meetings or from going to your doctor or therapist for help in losing weight.

**Blind Man's Bluff.** This saboteur specializes in making the dieter think that all her arduous dieting and deprivation aren't doing any good—so why not quit all this silly calorie-counting? The practitioner of Blind Man's Bluff often tells the dieter, "I can't see any difference," even though the dieter desperately needs some support and encouragement. Discouraged, the sabotaged dieter may quit and then blame herself.

**Guilt Giver.** This kind of saboteur gives emotionally rending ultimatums to the dieter. "If you loved me, you'd lose weight" is a classic Guilt Giver line. But the Guilt Giver only serves to increase feelings of guilt, instead of feelings of motivation and determination. Guilt-ridden, the dieter gets more and more anxious, and this usually culminates in going off the diet and onto a monumental high-calorie gorge.

**Freak Show/Martyrdom.** This saboteur eats normally or even overeats at the meals she shares with the family dieter. This makes the dieter feel like either a freak ("I'm the only one at the table who's eating cottage cheese and celery") or like a martyr ("Dear God, why do I have to be the only one at the table who's eating cottage cheese and celery").

Saboteurs who pull Freak Show/Martyrdom on dieters intensify the dieters' feelings of deprivation. And the more deprived you feel, the more anxious you are. And the more anxious you are, the more likely you are to succumb to the urge to overeat.

**Benedict Arnold.** This is a particularly nasty form of sabotage, which usually occurs between husband and wife.

The sabotaging spouse is literally traitorous. He or she attempts to use the children as tools, turning the kids against the overweight parent in an attempt to shame the heavy spouse. The ridicule of the children about Daddy's beer belly or Mommy's midriff bulge is supposed to shame the overweight person into weight loss. But more often, this shame turns to self-hate, which turns to overeating bouts. And the Benedict Arnold saboteur wins, not the dieter he or she is supposedly "helping."

The only defense against sabotage and self-sabotage is awareness. Be aware that you could defeat yourself. Or that your loved ones could defeat you, even as they claim to help you.

However, don't become unnecessarily paranoid about sabotage and self-sabotage. That would only be *another* way of sabotaging yourself.

Just be aware. And be wary.

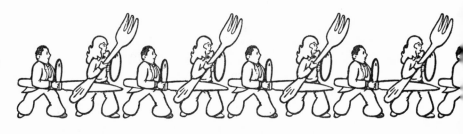

# 11 Do You Really Know When You're Hungry?

In discussing the reasons we can't get thin and stay that way, we've gone over the social, cultural, and emotional factors. But what about hunger? Isn't it hunger that makes us want to eat? Isn't it hunger that causes so many of us to break our diets?

The role of hunger is a factor in weight gain. But it's *not* the major reason we put on pounds. Most people—especially people with weight problems—don't really understand what hunger is. They mistake emotional states, such as fear, boredom, anger, and loneliness, for hunger. Other people confuse real hunger (the need to eat to maintain the body's functions) with mouth-hunger and tongue-hunger.

Both these hyphenated forms of hunger are real enough to the person experiencing them. You can recognize the presence of mouth-hunger when you feel a strong craving for something crunchy and chewy, a strong desire to bite into something. Tongue-hunger may be present when you have a strong desire for something soft and creamy, something that gets licked, something that gets explored with the tongue.

To varying degrees, compulsive/emotional eaters have lost touch with their own hunger. An experiment performed by psychiatrist Albert J. Stunkard of the University of Pennsylvania Hospital showed that obese people do not feel real hunger—at least, not in the same sense that people of normal weight do. Stunkard conducted his study by monitoring the stomach contractions of his subjects. When a stomach contracts, we experience a feeling of gnawing or of emptiness. This constitutes the almost indefinable hunger pang. Stunkard discovered that his obese experimental subjects didn't experience hunger when the monitoring devices showed that their stomachs were having hunger contractions.

Certainly, the obese subjects in Stunkard's study sometimes reported that they did feel hungry. But what they termed "hunger" didn't coincide with their stomachs' hunger contractions. These overweight people were out of touch with their own bodies' sensations. However, the normal-weight subjects in Stunkard's experiments could almost perfectly correlate their reports of "feeling hungry" with their stomachs' hunger contractions.

Stunkard's findings have been corroborated by other prominent obesity researchers. Dr. Hilde Bruch, a leading expert on eating disorders, noted that fat children don't seem to have learned—or to be able to learn—that there's a difference between hunger and various other "feeling states," such as tension, discomfort, and boredom. Psychologist Stanley Schachter performed other experiments that examined the relationship between the physiological *need* to eat (hunger) and the self-reported impulse to eat (false hunger). Schachter's work confirmed that overweight people are pretty much out of sync with the physiological signals that their bodies are sending out.

OK, so overweight people can't seem to identify real hunger as well as normal-weight or thin people can. But we still haven't answered the question—what is hunger? Scientists aren't in complete agreement about how hunger is triggered and felt by the body. One of the most compelling theories states that there's a "glucostat" in the hypothalamus section of the brain that monitors the levels of glucose (a kind of sugar) in the blood. This glucostat supposedly signals a warning—hunger—when glucose levels fall, thus telling us to eat.

Another theory says that there's a "lipostat" in the hypothalamus, which monitors levels of glycerol (a natural component of fat tissues) in the blood. When glycerol levels fall, the lipostat signals hunger. When glycerol levels rise sufficiently, the lipostat signals that you're full.

Still another hunger theory postulates that there's a thermostat in the brain that responds to fluctuations in the body temperature and in the temperature of the external environment. The thermostat theory holds that hunger is directly linked to minuscule changes in internal body temperature levels.

Another theory of hunger holds that an "aminostat" in the liver monitors the levels of amino acids in the body and signals hunger to the brain when supplies are depleted.

And finally, the trigeminal theory of hunger proposes that a nerve network located near the front of the cerebral hemispheres of the brain (the trigeminal) controls the hunger and feeding systems. This theory, formulated by Dr. H. Philip Zeigler, a research psychologist at the American Museum of Natural History, also accounts for the sensations of mouth-hunger and tongue-hunger that many of us experience. Zeigler believes that the oral sensations in the mouth and tongue may be important factors in arousing hunger. Thus, the smoothness of chocolate ice cream may contribute just as much to some people's overeating as does the dessert's sweet taste. Previously, it had been thought that the sweetness—not the texture experienced by the mouth and tongue—was the major culprit in triggering overeating.

No wonder you don't understand your own hunger—the scientists, as you've seen, can't agree on what hunger is either. All the theories of hunger listed above may have some elements of validity. Currently, the glucostat and lipostat theories are the more accepted. But all these hunger researchers have one area of accord—it's not your stomach that tells you you're hungry, it's your brain.

Yes, the brain is the principal arbiter of both hunger and satiety (fullness). But the part of the brain that triggers hunger is not the conscious, logical upper brain of the cerebral cortex. The part of the brain that tells us we're hungry is probably a portion of the hypothalamus, a more primitive part of the brain that developed much further back in human and animal evolution.

The hypothalamus operates on the unconscious, autonomic level. But its commands to the body are potent, nonetheless. Researchers have demonstrated this by inflicting damage or lesions to groups of cells in the presumed "hunger center" of the hypothalamus. The damage sometimes resulted in the experimental animals acquiring a drive to eat voraciously until they became obese. Or the damage could result in complete apathy toward food, leading to severe weight loss. It's thought that amphetamine-based weight-reducing drugs also work by affecting cells in the hypothalamus's hunger center, perhaps temporarily short-circuiting them.

Hunger can be satisfied by remarkably little food, if what you mean by hunger is hunger pangs (specifically, the stomach contractions). A third of a banana, for instance, will stop the stomach contractions. But the feeling of hunger itself won't disappear until a change in the bloodstream's glucose or glycerol levels (depending on your hunger theory) affects specific cell groups in the brain. Thus, the brain is still the ultimate judge of whether you're hungry or full.

Different people show markedly different responses to hunger. Some people are impelled to eat by the first little twinge of hunger that they experience. Other people actually enjoy feeling hunger. They associate it with getting thin or with being in complete, stoic control of themselves. These are the types who say, "A little hunger never hurt anybody. Builds the character to resist it."

Some people eat in anticipation of their hunger. They're actually afraid that if they feel hungry, "something awful might happen." This is the kind of person who casually mentions, while wolfing down a Big Mac, "I'm not actually hungry. I just ate an hour ago, but I know I won't have a chance to eat again until pretty late this evening, so I'd better fill up now."

And then there is the majority of the overweight, who can never identify or experience real physiological hunger at all.

## THE HUNGER-AWARENESS PROGRAM

If you're one of the last two groups, perhaps you should embark upon a brief program of hunger-awareness exercises. As long as you are in reasonably good health, these hunger-awareness techniques will not adversely affect you. If you do become dizzy or faint, sucking on half an orange or eating half a banana will probably correct this momentary reaction. And you can continue with your experiencing of hunger as if nothing had happened.

1. Here's the first hunger-awareness exercise: delay eating your dinner by at least two hours. If you normally eat at 6:00 P.M., postpone dining until 8:00 P.M. The delay in eating your main meal should not be considered part of a diet. It's just a way of getting in touch with your personal way of experiencing hunger. Pay attention to your body. What signals is it giving you? Is your stomach rumbling or growling? Do you feel an emptiness or a gnawing deep in the pit of your midsection? Does your throat, perhaps, feel achey?

Any of these reactions might be your personal hunger response. Or you may experience hunger quite differently. The important thing right now is to *feel* the hunger, so that you can recognize real, physiological hunger in the future. Don't be afraid of the hunger. Don't run from it. Feel it. Examine your body's sensations carefully. Use this delaying-eating tactic to get to know yourself better, in this one small way.

• • •

2. The next hunger-awareness exercise progresses a little deeper into the nature of hunger. This time experience hunger by skipping a meal. The point now is to examine the nature of your hunger as the hours pass. Let's say you're skipping lunch. Do you feel hungrier and hungrier all afternoon long, until dinner? Or does your hunger taper off? Or does your hunger ebb and flow like the tides?

Also, pay particular attention to your emotional reactions to skipping a meal. Do you feel deprived, scared, resentful, noble? Try to tell the difference between your emotional reactions and real physiological hunger. Remember, all your emotions do not automatically transfer into hunger pangs. You can consciously override these feelings now that you know what your genuine hunger reaction is.

3. After you've done the skipping-a-meal exercise two or three times, you might want to progress to the third level of hunger-awareness exercises. This time, don't eat all day long. For one whole day, give your stomach a rest. Again, don't embark on this voluntary fast in order to lose weight. This isn't a diet. This is an exercise in self-knowledge and self-awareness. If you feel dizzy or faint, remember, you can usually revive yourself quickly by drinking a glass of orange juice or by sucking on half an orange or by eating half a small banana. This isn't supposed to be a torture. It's supposed to be a means of modest self-discovery.

On this brief fast, you aren't going to get a spiritual high. But you will probably get a few hunger pangs, or maybe you'll get a lot of them. Examine your reaction to these feelings of hunger.

How do you react to your hunger emotionally? Are you scared or proud—or what? Do you find yourself during this day wanting to eat more because of emotional triggers? For instance, your boss yells at you; you feel nobody loves you; you hate the way you look.

Maybe you'll find yourself wanting to eat because of physiological reasons: "God, I'm starving!" Don't cheat by chewing gum or swallowing quarts of diet soft drinks to give yourself a bloated feeling, so that you'll never approach feelings of hunger.

Feel your anxiety levels rise as you skip breakfast, lunch, and dinner. Notice how your anxiety levels and your feelings of real physiological hunger are not the same thing after all. That's a discovery. And that's why you're fasting for one day: to get in touch with your real hungers.

You may find, after this final hunger-awareness exercise, that you hunger more for love, attention, excitement, or security than you hunger for food. It's an intriguing distinction, one that naturally thin people seem to be born with the capacity to make. But it's a distinction that people with weight problems seem to have to *learn*.

Now that you understand hunger a little better, you might be interested in satiety. This refers to the feeling of fullness, of having eaten enough. All the theories of physiological hunger assume that once the temperature or the glucose, glycerol, or amino-acid level rises sufficiently, the brain's hunger center will turn off its hunger signals. This turn-off is satiety.

University of Texas psychologist Devandra Singh found that once their hunger is aroused, obese people find it harder to shut down/turn off their hunger drives than thin or normal-weight people do. But if the food tastes bad enough, even the obese are found to feel full rather quickly. In this way, taste can be a powerful regulator of food intake.

Conversely, when a food tastes truly delicious, it's harder to feel satiated and to stop eating. This reaction to delicious food is virtually the same for both the thin and the overweight.

Of course, there are many people who will eat (and overeat) just because a food is exceptionally tasty: "I'm really full, but I'll sure make room for some of that coconut cream pie."

Taste works along with hunger in helping us to regulate our consumption of food. Taste was especially vital to our prehistoric ancestors, who spent most of their time and energy searching for food. These early men could use taste as a safety factor in deciding whether or not to eat foods they found growing wild. The primitive man might have found berries that looked succulent, for instance, but if a small taste showed him the berries were bitter or bad-tasting, then he wouldn't swallow more. This reaction to bad-tasting foods probably saved many of our ancestors from eating unwholesome or decaying foods and from accidental poisoning as well.

For a sense that has been so much discussed and relied on throughout human history, taste is curiously limited. Studies have determined that human beings respond to only four taste qualities: salt, sour, sweet, and bitter. The difference in taste between a pot roast and an avocado lies in varying concentrations and combinations of these four tastes and also depends on where the food strikes your tongue. The taste buds at the tip of the tongue, for example, are more sensitive to sweet flavors, the sides to sour, and the back of the tongue to bitter. Taste isn't a "pure" sense. It's a melange of sensations of texture, temperature, and smell.

Yet taste is one of the very first senses to develop in humans after birth. Tests have demonstrated that even premature babies can tell the difference between sweet and salty flavors. Another study showed that even during the first day of life, a full-term infant will prefer sugar water to plain, unflavored water. Thus, it seems, we naturally seek out sweets. Your rampant sweet tooth has a firm biological basis, quite apart from your cultural conditioning that sweets are desirable and delectable.

Even the "jaded palate," which would seem to be a cultural product of increased sophistication, has a biological basis. The probable cause of the jaded palate is that, after age forty-five, there's a decline in the number of functioning taste buds in most individuals. Since they can literally taste less, they find that food no longer seems quite as appealing. The loss of taste buds with age is a contributing factor to the apathy toward food that many elderly people experience.

Most tastes, as we discussed in earlier chapters, are culturally determined. The culture in which you are raised dictates to you what should and should not taste "good." That's why Indians from Kerala province think lobster and prawns taste bad, while Europeans pay good money to import the same tasty Kerala lobsters and prawns that the natives shun.

Since taste is culturally determined, a person without conditioning in his host culture's likes and dislikes might pick food combinations far from the natives' norm. That's the reason we laugh at one of the running jokes on television's "Mork and Mindy," in which Mork, the alien being from outer space, loves to eat bologna sundaes. Culturally conditioned, we "know" that bologna and ice cream taste bad together, even though we have probably never tried that taste combination.

But even within fairly uniform cultural concepts of what tastes good and what tastes bad, individuals have their own idiosyncratic variations. We have a taste for something, a craving for it, which seems irrational, but which is possibly caused by our personality structure.

For instance, people who are "sensation-seekers" may use their taste sensations to avoid boredom. Sensation-seekers search for intense, often risky experiences in their daily lives; they're people who enjoy skydiving, downhill skiing, auto racing, and other dangerous hobbies. So naturally these sensation-seekers prefer chewy foods, instead of soft; spicy foods, instead of bland; and bitter foods, instead of sweets, according to research done by Dr. Marvin Zuckerman, director of clinical psychology programs at the University of Delaware. "These people crave extremes in taste, not the usual pap of American food—soft white bread and that sort of thing," Zuckerman says.

Of course, not everyone is a sensation-seeker; others seek love or security from their foods. Dr. Benjamin Belden, head of the Gestalt Institute of the Chicago Center for Behavior Modification, found in his clinical practice that "obese people prefer mushy foods. Eating a lot can also be a substitute for aggression. You take another bite of a chewy or crunchy food, instead of turning and biting what's bothering you."

Several years ago, the U.S. Department of Defense (DOD) made a study of the food preferences of enlisted men. The object was to see if there was a relationship between diet and personality traits. A test group of soldiers was encouraged to select whatever they wanted to eat from a group of 150 foods. The DOD's month-long study resulted in some fascinating correlations between the foods the experimental subjects preferred and their personality types. For instance:

• Meat eaters are officer types. They're enthusiastic, like action, and enjoy selling themselves, ideas, and products.

• People who prefer fish, fruits, and vegetables for their meals tend to prefer books, music, and art in their recreation hours. They're not highly competitive and tend to be somewhat shy in social situations.

• If you relish starchy foods like rice, mashed potatoes, and spaghetti, you're probably rather complacent. You may avoid making hard decisions or judgments.

• People who prefer eating salads are fast-moving types. They speak slightly faster, move faster, and work faster than those who prefer other food groups. They're also generally sympathetic and are willing to listen to their friends' and associates' problems.

• If you are very fond of dairy products (particularly milk, yogurt, and ice cream), you may be displaying through your food preferences a basic insecurity in your personality structure. Choosing these foods often indicates a desire to return to Mother and to childhood days.

• Finally, the kind of people who like desserts above all are an excellent officer type, the DOD found. That's because the dessert-eaters usually like to dominate any situation.

If the DOD study is correct, there's a definite link between your personality type and the kinds of foods you crave. However, other researchers believe that food yens can be physiological in origin. They think that unusual cravings

186

and strange tastes in your mouth may be early signs of disease.

A loss of taste sensations or a sudden dislike for the taste of meat can be an early indicator of cancer, according to Dr. Robert I. Henkin of the Georgetown University Medical Center. Henkin found that loss of taste can often be linked to undetected brain tumors and tumors of the gastrointestinal tract. The symptom of having a bad taste in your mouth also may be connected to stomach cancer. "In some patients, one of the earliest signs of cancer is that meat tastes terrible," Henkin noted. "Lung, ovarian, and breast tumors, too, can cause loss of appetite and changes in perceptions of taste and smell."

One New York City internist and nutrition expert, Dr. Robert Giller, theorizes that taste sensations can signal many medical problems. A sour taste in the mouth or a craving for sour foods and drinks (for example, lemons) can indicate liver or gall-bladder problems, Giller believes. A bitter taste in the mouth or a craving for bitter foods can be connected to colitis or a vitamin and mineral deficiency caused by intestinal malfunction. And a constant desire for spicy, highly flavored foods can point to lung or sinus troubles. People who smoke a lot also lose their sense of taste to some degree, and Giller found that they, too, crave spicy foods.

What do all these divergent theories of taste preferences tell us? Basically, that our yens and cravings for certain foods don't just come out of thin air. These desires often have psychological or physiological foundations. And by paying attention to our food cravings and tastes, we can gain new insights into our emotional and physical functioning.

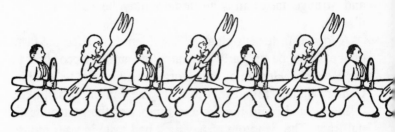

# 12  The Best Diet for You

All diets work.

No diets work.

Both of the above statements are true, even though they contradict each other. How can this be so?

All diets work, because any system of caloric deprivation (consuming fewer calories than your body needs to function) will be effective—at first. If you change your eating habits drastically on a diet—plunge down to only 800 calories a day when you're used to 3,000 or eliminate almost all carbohydrates when you're used to eating lots of breads and sweets—you will, of course, lose weight initially, if only because you're eating a lot less than you formerly did or because you're limiting your dietary choices, totally deleting food groups like starches and sweets that formerly supplied many of your daily calories.

When people change their eating patterns abruptly, they generally tend to eat less. That's why all diets work. But these drastic changes in eating habits usually can't be maintained over the long haul. Enthusiasm for the diet wanes, or you simply experience an uncontrollable urge to binge. And so that diet, once successful for you, fails in the long run. You can't stick to that diet forever; you can't make it into a new way of life for yourself. Why? Because eating habits and patterns are inordinately hard to alter once you're an adult or even an adolescent. And that's why the statement "No diets work" is also true. Because about 90 percent of all successful dieters—people who have lost ten pounds or more—will eventually turn into failed dieters. They will regain the weight they've so arduously lost within two years. Often these once successful dieters will gain back even more weight than they originally lost on their diets, putting them in even worse shape (literally and figuratively) than they were in to begin with.

As Dr. Theodore van Itallie, director of the obesity research program at New York's St. Luke's Hospital, explains, "There is no particular diet with which you can achieve *permanent* weight loss." In order to keep pounds off permanently, Dr. van Itallie says, "you must change your pattern of lifetime eating. You must also change your behavior and eating habits. The way to keep weight off for good should be by learning to balance energy intake and expenditure."

Put in simpler terms, if you want to lose weight and keep it off, learn to eat fewer calories than your body needs to perform its daily functions. Use up the calories you ingest. Sounds simple, doesn't it? But it's fiendishly hard to put this kind of solid, sensible advice into practice.

That's why so many people end up on crash diets. They drastically reduce their caloric intake, sometimes down to 500 calories a day. This produces speedy weight loss. But *nobody* should stay on a crash diet indefinitely—to do that would result in severe nutritional imbalances and possible injury to the dieter's health. So everybody winds up breaking their crash diets sooner or later. They feel guilty for their lack of willpower. But what's really happening is that their bodies are acting wisely by forcing these crash dieters to take in more calories and more varied foods before they cause themselves permanent physical harm.

Crash diets inevitably lead to failure in permanent weight loss, though they may, at first, seem to work. The crash diets are overly restrictive of the kinds of foods that may be eaten and of the number of calories that may be consumed daily.

One popular, typical crash diet is called the Cottage Cheese and Grapefruit Diet. This consists of only 600 calories a day (the average adult male needs 2,400 calories a day; the average adult female needs 2,000 calories a day). The 600 calories on this crash diet are limited to only two types of food, cottage cheese (the low-fat diet variety) and grapefruit. The person on the Cottage Cheese and Grapefruit Diet eats six small meals a day, consisting of one-fourth of a cup of cottage cheese and half a grapefruit. The dieter is also advised to drink plenty of water, and, if he's really starving, to add low-calorie foods like lettuce, mushrooms, and celery.

On a crash diet like this, food intake is so severely restricted that the earnest dieter will wind up with a deficiency of vital vitamins and minerals. He will probably feel weak, dizzy, even faint. But he will lose weight. Which he'll promptly regain after going off the crash diet.

Because crash diets are overly restrictive, they lead the dieter into severe feelings of deprivation, both psychological and physical. This leads to breaking the crash diet. It also leads to guilt, self-recrimination, and feelings of failure and inadequacy.

## FAD DIETS CAN BE HAZARDOUS TO YOUR HEALTH

Some crash and fad diets can actually kill you. Over a dozen deaths have been attributed directly to overzealous following of the so-called "liquid protein diet." The prepared liquid protein (made from predigested collagen) which people on this diet buy does not contain a proper balance of amino acids (the building blocks of proteins), nor is it usually adequately fortified with minerals, according to Dr. Myron Winick, director of the Columbia University Institute of Human Nutrition. Because of these deficiencies, the liquid protein diet can actually be harder on the dieter's body than total starvation, Winick believes. The lack of potassium in the liquid protein diet can lead to fatigue, dizziness, even sudden death.

The liquid protein diet is especially danger-fraught for people with metabolic, kidney, liver, blood vessel, and heart diseases. The liquid protein diet has been blamed for side effects ranging from bad breath and constipation to dizziness and cardiac arrest.

Low-carbohydrate diets seem less harmful than the liquid protein regime, but they also have their hazards. Low-carbohydrate diets are popularly called by many names, such as the drinking man's diet, the Air Force diet, the Stillman water diet, the Atkins diet, and the calories-don't-count diet. These diets produce an immediate weight loss, since all or nearly all sugars and starches are eliminated from the dieter's consumption. That means few or no vegetables, fruits, grains, breads, or sweets.

However, a considerable portion of the weight loss in the early stages of these diets is from water loss, not from actual fat loss. So once the dieter starts eating carbohydrates again, the body starts retaining water again, and those water-loss pounds are regained.

Ketosis is another highly undesirable, even hazardous result of these low-carbohydrate miracle diets. Ketosis occurs when the body, lacking carbohydrates, burns fats for energy. But these fats are burned incompletely, which leads to a tremendous increase in the number of ketone compounds present in the blood and urine. Ketosis can cause fatigue and dizziness, nausea and vomiting, mental daze and low blood pressure. It can also produce kidney failure in persons with kidney disease.

Physicians cite other hazards of low-carbohydrate diets, ranging from excessive uric acid in the blood (which can lead to gout), disturbances in heart rhythm, defective brain development in fetuses carried by pregnant low-carbohydrate dieters, and complications leading to uremic poisoning. Without fruits and vegetables in sufficient quantity, people on low-carbohydrate, high-protein diets have also been found to suffer from scurvy (caused by vitamin C deficiency) and even from loss of bone (caused by calcium deficiency).

It seems like a rather high price to pay in order to lose a few pounds.

## DEBUNKING DRUGS FOR DIETING

Diet pills have been frequently prescribed by doctors to aid their patients' weight loss. The trouble is that diet pills are dangerous, harmful, and useless. Most diet pills are really amphetamines. They cut the dieter's appetite dramatically at first, but their effect on appetite generally wears off in a few weeks. If the dieter persists in taking amphetamines, she may grow nervous and edgy, and have difficulty sleeping. Prolonged use of amphetamines can lead to psychological addiction to these drugs. Many of the so-called speed freaks of the sixties drug culture got their start by copping a few of their mothers' diet pills. The results were disastrous for the speed freaks. And the results are still disastrous for many frustrated dieters who turn to amphetamines as a last-ditch way of shedding excess pounds. In response to this widespread abuse of amphetamines, the U.S. Food and Drug Administration in 1979 proposed a ban on doctors' prescribing such pills for dieting and appetite suppression.

Amphetamines are no good for you. If you go to a doctor who prescribes amphetamines for weight loss, do not fill the prescription. Do not take the diet pills. Seek out another doctor who can guide you in weight loss *without amphetamines.* If your friends or family are taking amphetamines for weight-loss reasons, encourage them to stop taking these harmful drugs. The side effects of amphetamines and the possibilities of slipping into drug abuse and even addiction are not worth the slight possibility of losing a few pounds through amphetamine-induced loss of appetite. As the drug culture used to put it, "Speed kills." And it could kill *you.*

There are other drugs that unscrupulous or ignorant doctors have prescribed in weight-loss regimes that you should know about—and avoid.

Diuretics (commonly called "water pills") don't help you lose fat; all they do is eliminate pounds of water from your body. Once you stop taking the diuretics, you'll regain those "water pounds." Prolonged or careless use of diuretics can seriously deplete your body's stores of potassium and sodium. These deficiencies, in turn, can result in nausea, fatigue, dizziness, and weakness.

Human chorionic gonadotropin (commonly called HCG) has been used in quacks' weight-loss regimes in the form of daily or weekly injections of HCG, combined with a 500-calorie-a-day diet. Naturally, people lose weight on this program. Not because of the effects of the HCG (which is derived from the urine of pregnant females) but because of the minimal caloric intake. Medical researchers have found no connection between HCG and weight loss, and the safety of HCG ingestion has never been verified.

Again, if you are going to a doctor who wants to place you on an HCG-injection weight-loss program, don't go through with this drug "therapy." Find yourself another doctor—for your health's sake.

Thyroid hormone has also been injected into dieters to promote weight loss. The trouble is that medical researchers say thyroid injections are "ineffective" in producing permanent weight loss. Unless you have a genuine thyroid condition (i.e., hypothyroidism), injections of thyroid hormone could be hazardous to your health. The injections could seriously upset the hormonal balance of a dieter with normal thyroid function. Thyroid injections are particularly ill-advised for people with heart disease.

OK, you say. Amphetamines are bad for me. HCG is bad for me. Thyroid injections are bad for me. Diuretics don't really help. And crash diets work in the short term but fail dismally in the long run. What can a person do if he really wants to lose pounds permanently?

## THE BEST DIET

The best diet for people in generally good health is the Sensible 1200 Diet. It consists of 1,200 calories a day, safely and effectively divided among the four major food groups. "This is the safest and best weight-loss diet that exists today," according to American Medical Association nutritionist H. Louise Dillon. This diet, unlike crash and fad diets, contains all the nutrients recommended for optimum human health maintenance by the Food and Nutrition Board of the National Research Council.

The Sensible 1200 Diet will result in a weight loss of one to two pounds per week, depending on the individual. This is a gradual weight loss, but it will have relatively few unpleasant side effects like the nausea and weakness of ketosis.

The Sensible 1200 Diet also allows you to express your own personal food preferences in the diet, to some extent. You make up your own diet each day by following a few easy steps.

1. *You must select your foods from each of the four major food groups,* and you must eat all the required portions of these foods every day, in order to maintain nutritional balance.

● *From the Milk Foods Group: two portions daily.* You can take these in the form of two eight-ounce glasses of milk (skimmed milk is preferred because it's lower in calories) or buttermilk. Or else you can have two portions daily from other milk products, such as cheese, cottage cheese, or yogurt.

● *From the Vegetables and Fruits Food Group: four portions daily.* Eat at least one portion of high-vitamin-C food every day; good choices are citrus fruits, broccoli, and tomatoes. Three or four times a week, you should include a yellow fruit or a deep yellow vegetable (squash, carrots) or a dark green leafy vegetable.

● *From the Meat and Protein Foods Group: at least two*

*portions daily*. Choose from fish, poultry, meats, eggs, and cheeses. Nonanimal sources of proteins include nuts, peanut butter, dried beans, and peas. Try to eat one portion of liver weekly.

● *From the Cereal and Grain Foods Group: four portions daily*. This food group includes breads, cereals (preferably eat only low- or no-sugar prepared cereals), pasta, noodles, rice, grits, corn meal, and baked goods. Wholegrain foods are the best choice in this group.

2. *Limit yourself to 1,200 calories a day for women, 1,600 calories a day for men*. You must eat the number of recommended portions from each food group *every day*. But you must also keep track of how many calories you're eating of these permissible foods. You can buy a low-priced calorie-counter book to keep track of your calories. Don't go crazy counting calories, but do use your calorie-counter book to keep yourself from going overboard on high-calorie meats, breads and cereals, and cheeses.

3. *Don't add sugar* to your foods or beverages. Don't add cream to your coffee; try to stick to skimmed milk. Don't think that honey is permissible when sugar is not. Avoid soft drinks and other beverages with sugar.

The Sensible 1200 Diet is based on an "anti-coronary" diet devised in the late fifties by Dr. Norman Jolliffe, in conjunction with the Bureau of Nutrition of the New York City Health Department. When Jean Nidetch was an overweight housewife, she went on Dr. Jolliffe's diet plan to lose weight. Later, Nidetch used a modified version of the Jolliffe diet as the basis of the original eating program for Weight Watchers, the weight-loss organization that she founded.

For maximum success in long-term weight loss, it's best to personalize your own Sensible 1200 Diet, using the foods in the basic food groups that please your personal palate the most. But to help you in constructing your personalized Sensible 1200 Diet days, here are two possible menu plans, each totaling about 1,200 calories. Men can add 400 calories a day to total about 1,600 calories.

*Sample Menu 1*

Breakfast—4 oz. orange juice

1 scrambled egg

1 slice whole wheat toast

1 pat butter or margarine

8 oz. skimmed milk or buttermilk

coffee or tea

Lunch—4 oz. vegetable soup

3 to 4 oz. tuna fish

2 tsp. diet mayonnaise

lettuce, celery, and cucumber salad (as much as desired), with vinegar or lemon juice as dressing

2 slices rye bread (toasted or untoasted)

carrot sticks (as many as desired)

1 oz. Swiss cheese

coffee or tea

Dinner—4 to 6 oz. baked or broiled chicken

1 half-cup serving broccoli

1 half-cup serving baked acorn squash

hearts of lettuce salad (as much as desired), with vinegar or lemon juice as dressing

½ cup macaroni or other noodles

¼ of a whole cantaloupe

coffee or tea

Snack—8 oz. skimmed milk or buttermilk

4 oz. fresh strawberries

*Sample Menu 2*

Breakfast—½ grapefruit

4 oz. cooked cereal

4 oz. skimmed milk

coffee or tea

Lunch—ham and cheese sandwich, made with 1 slice
ham, 1 slice American or Swiss cheese, lettuce
leaves, 1 pat butter, 2 slices whole wheat bread
(toasted or untoasted)

assorted crudités (carrots, celery, radishes)

1 whole peach or orange

4 oz. skimmed milk

coffee or tea

Dinner—6 oz. baked, broiled, or poached fish

8 spears asparagus

tossed green salad (as much as desired),
with vinegar or lemon juice as dressing

1 slice toast

½ cup fresh cherries

coffee or tea

Snack—4 oz. skimmed milk

melon or other fruit, 1 serving

no-sugar soft drink (as much as desired)

## THE ULTIMATE DIET

The Sensible 1200 Diet is a very good diet, but it is not the
Ultimate Diet. The Ultimate Diet cannot be found in books
or magazine articles. The Ultimate Diet is a personalized
diet plan that combines regimes for weight loss and weight
maintenance. This personalized eating program should be
tailor-made for you by a certified nutritionist. You can find
a reputable nutritionist by referral from your family doctor. Or you can phone your local hospital or university
medical school and ask for the names of staff nutritionists
who accept private patients.

When you consult your nutritionist, you should discuss

what foods you like, what foods you detest, what special weight-loss problems you have. The nutritionist should then be able to help you in designing a weight-loss program that is sane, sensible, and effective.

Why should your weight-loss program be tailor-made? Because no two people lose weight in precisely the same way.

It's not widely publicized, but it is a medical fact that on the same dietary regime, the same number of calories, the same foods, some dieters will lose weight; some dieters will maintain the same weight; and some dieters will gain weight! No, this isn't fair, but it is the way different bodies use food, metabolize it, and burn up fuel.

A trained nutritionist can help you to compensate for your body's idiosyncrasies in burning up food fuels and losing weight. Creating a personalized weight-loss diet will allow you to diet with maximum benefits, maximum weight reduction, and minimum negative side effects.

However, when you consult a nutritionist, don't just focus on weight loss. This is an excellent opportunity to learn about healthful *lifelong* eating habits. You won't— or shouldn't—be on a diet all your life. For those times when you're eating "normally," a nutritionist-devised eating plan can help you stay healthy and keep excess pounds off.

## MINDPOWER BOOSTS ANY DIET

Willpower usually gets defeated by wantpower—"I want a candy bar" or "I want a piece of cheesecake" or "I want a plate of fettucine Alfredo." But you can use your mindpower to help boost your willpower, your resolve to stay on a diet.

The first way you can employ mindpower is to decide on a deep mental level that you *do* want to lose weight, that you *do* want to stay on a diet, that you *do* have everything to gain by losing. Get your mind to help your body. Your thought processes, your attitudes toward dieting, can help ensure success in weight loss and weight maintenance.

The most effective use of mindpower is in changing your

life-style. If you go on a diet, but keep thinking about the day you can go off it, the day you can overeat again, then you're doomed to gain back any and all weight you lose. But you can change your mind to change your life-style, and this can virtually guarantee weight maintenance.

Certain mental techniques will increase your mindpower in the direction of changing to a less food-oriented life-style.

Hypnosis is one frequently used method of increasing the desire to lose weight and of decreasing the psychological bases of your appetite. Hypnosis has been used with some success in breaking many bad habits like smoking, nail-biting, and overeating. When you consult a qualified hypnotherapist, he or she will instruct you in how to place yourself in a hypnotic state. After a few visits (sometimes one visit is sufficient), you will be able to practice autosuggestion (self-hypnosis) for weight control.

But for self-hypnosis to succeed, you must *want* to lose weight. You must be willing to practice the self-hypnosis techniques your hypnotherapist has taught you, and this involves using self-hypnosis daily, even several times each day. This requires motivation—that's essential for hypnosis to be effective.

Hypnotherapy is not a parlor trick. Qualified hypnotherapists are usually physicians (often psychiatrists) or clinical psychologists. *Don't* go to a hypnotist who performs parlor magic tricks with hypnotism or who advertises. You can locate a *qualified* hypnotherapist in your area by sending a stamped, self-addressed envelope to the American Society of Clinical Hypnosis, 2400 E. Devon Avenue, Suite 218, Des Plaines, Illinois 60018. Or you may write to the Society for Clinical and Experimental Hypnosis, Inc., 129A King's Park Drive, Liverpool, New York 13088; remember to include a stamped, self-addressed envelope here, too.

Techniques for autosuggestion are also taught at the Silva Mind Control centers located in many major American cities. The Silva techniques focus on positive thinking, positive self-image, and habit control in general, not just in terms of weight loss. Instruction in autosuggestion is part of a four-day general self-improvement and self-actualization course. Silva Mind Control does not seek to control other people's minds; the object is to help you learn to control your own mind and, thus, your own life.

For some people, the more spiritual disciplines of **meditation** and **yoga** aid greatly in weight reduction and weight maintenance. Some dieters use meditation as a method of calming the inner tensions and outer stresses that lead to bouts of overeating. Yoga, of course, focuses on the union of mind and body. Hatha yoga is the form of yoga that concentrates on physical exercises, as well as meditation, to achieve a new, more calm and centered life-style for its practitioners. Yoga is taught in most major American cities by both Indian spiritual teachers and American secular instructors at such unlikely places as YMCAs.

If hypnosis and yoga strike you as too exotic, you may choose to rely on a more scientific method of boosting your dieting mindpower. Behavior modification has been used with striking success, particularly in the weight-loss program conducted at the University of Pennsylvania Medical School in Philadelphia. The Pennsylvania behavior-modification program has resulted in successes of up to 30 percent of its dieters (meaning that the dieters kept off the weight they lost for at least two years).

The principles of behavior modification derive in large part from behavioral psychology and its concepts of operant conditioning. In laymen's terms, behavior modification is the restructuring of your eating habits so that they work *for* your weight loss, instead of against it. In behavior modification programs, the small components of eating behavior are broken down, analyzed, and then consciously changed by the dieter.

Here's an example of behavior modification techniques. It is known that the slower you eat, the less food it takes to satisfy your hunger pangs. This is because it takes twenty minutes from the time food is ingested until the satiety response occurs. To take advantage of this satiety effect, your behavior-modification plan might feature ways in which you would learn to eat more slowly. For instance, you might be instructed to put your fork down between each bite of food. You might be asked to chew your food more carefully, instead of quickly gulping it down. Small changes, yes—but many such changes may lead to significant weight loss.

Another way in which behavior modification commonly uses time to cut down calorie consumption is achieved by having the dieter keep a log of her eating patterns. She writes down what she eats, at what hours of the day. By looking back at a week's carefully kept chart, the dieter will see that clear eating patterns emerge. She may overeat late at night, for instance, while her eating habits during the rest of the day are good. So to achieve weight loss, behavior modification principles would go into play: the dieter would be told to eat normally all day long—except during those late-night hours when she usually binges. This requires less willpower than calorie-cutting all day long, and yet could result in about the same degree of weight loss. The calorie-cutting is focused, instead of diffused painfully over an entire day and night.

Another mindpower method related to behavior modification is **aversion therapy**. In this method, the dieter is taught to associate foods with unpleasant experiences or with distasteful objects. Let's say a dieter frequently overeats one specific food, such as apple pie. Using aversion therapy, the dieter is instructed to look at the apple pie before eating it and imagine that cockroaches are crawling all over the apple slices. This is such a disgusting image that most dieters would lose their desire for apple pie in short order. Repeated use of this kind of aversion imagery could create a permanent dislike for apple pie or any other high-calorie, high-temptation food that spells this particular dieter's caloric downfall.

Aversion therapy works by being intentionally disgusting. So be forewarned, it's not for the faint-hearted or for those whose motivation is shaky.

If you choose either behavior modification or aversion

therapy, seek out a qualified therapist, preferably a psychiatrist or clinical psychologist. Good behavior modification programs can sometimes be found at university-related hospitals and medical schools. Try not to patronize unqualified people who practice so-called behavior-modification techniques at reducing clinics and exercise studios. They may do you more harm than good. Don't entrust your mind to anyone unless you're convinced he or she is thoroughly qualified, professional, and competent.

To succeed permanently at weight loss and weight maintenance, some changes must be made in your life-style. You must find other things to do besides eat to reward, comfort, and console yourself. The next chapter gives you 121 things to do besides consuming calories—activities designed to boost your dieting power.

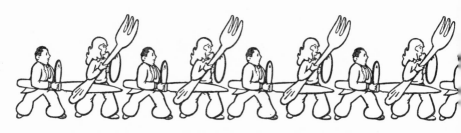

# 13 Instead of Eating: Or, 121 Things to Do Instead of Stuffing Your Face

By now, you've learned many of the reasons that you eat and overeat. But you also have to put that new knowledge into practice to help yourself. When the compulsion to overeat strikes, you must have a strategy prepared to avert a food binge. One of the reasons the urge to overeat occurs is that we use food—eating—to camouflage our true feelings. Instead of venting anger, instead of expressing dissatisfaction or boredom, we eat—and eat and eat. Thus, one of the strategies you should take to conquer a fat attack is to unleash your emotions, feel your feelings.

A second important reason for overeating is that people who tend to turn toward eating for comfort, pleasure, reward, and entertainment have a limited repertoire of behavior. Their response to any emotion—sorrow or joy—is to eat. If you're prone to emotional overeating, you have to learn other things to do that are just as satisfying, perhaps even more satisfying, than eating. You must learn to connect with your other senses, so that something other than food will give you pleasure. You must learn to revel in the senses of touch, sight, hearing, even smell.

When you're trying to find something to do with yourself

instead of eating, it helps to classify these noneating sources of gratification into basic strategy groups:

1. Nonfattening oral activities that serve as substitutes for eating

2. Anxiety-reducing activities

3. Ways to increase your range of *pleasurable* activities (Don't let guilt spoil your enjoyment of these newfound pleasures. You *deserve* pleasure.)

4. Body awareness activities (By learning to enjoy your body more, to feel more integrated with your body, you'll presumably increase your sensitivity to your body's needs. And that means you may eat less to keep your body healthier and feeling better.)

5. Desperation strategies. When all else fails and self-control seems a fantasy, do something with your hands and/or mouth so that eating is impossible. This means that you'll get yourself in a place (shower stall) or position (hands smeared with dirt from gardening) or situation (attending a lecture) where eating is virtually unthinkable.

Here's a list of 121 things to do instead of stuffing your face. These strategies can actually work for you, but you'll have to personalize your own eating-avoidance methods. You can do this by running over this list and checking off the items that appeal to your unique personality type and interests. The crucial step comes next.

Don't merely check off an anti-eating activity. Get up *now* and get the necessary equipment to do it. This may involve buying a needlework project and placing it prominently in the kitchen as an alternative—a genuine, not imagined, alternative—to opening the refrigerator. Or you may have to go out and buy athletic equipment or playing cards or even bubble bath.

The important thing is to prepare in advance for your next fat attack. Have your anti-eating activities listed clearly on a card or slip of paper. Keep one copy in your wallet and another copy on the refrigerator door. Make certain that your anti-eating strategy equipment is readily available—no rummaging through closets or drawers. If you delay in putting one of these strategies into action, the compulsion to eat/overeat may become too strong to resist or to avoid.

At the very least, these 121 strategies should give you some concrete ideas, so that next time you'll be the conqueror of your fat attack, not its victim.

1. Talk—to a friend, on the phone, into a tape recorder.

2. Write. This is a good substitute for the oral satisfaction of talking. You can write something creative (poems, stories, skits) or you can keep a diarylike journal to express your feelings in some way other than eating.

3. Try little-calorie oralities. These could include chewing sugar-free gum, sucking sugar-free mints or candies, gnawing on a piece of rubber or a pencil, sucking ice cubes.

4. Try a no-calorie orality—sing or hum.

5. Take up a musical instrument, particularly one that involves a lot of mouth work. The instrument will be something you can shove into your mouth, so that you can't shove food in at the same time. Some "mouth-heavy" instruments include the harmonica (easy enough for even the least musical individuals), flute, saxophone, clarinet, trumpet, recorder (also rather easy), bagpipes (especially if you're Irish or Scottish—ethnic-pride time), pennywhistle, trombone, tuba.

6. Read aloud. You don't necessarily need an audience; you can just read to yourself out loud. Practice your diction. Try out different accents, just for fun. Act out emotions or scenes from stories and plays. You can express yourself without embarrassment, because you're alone.

7. A more offbeat no-calorie orality—learn bird calls.

8. Kiss. This no-calorie orality temporarily prevents you from eating and tones facial muscles, besides making you and your loved ones feel special.

9. Clean your house. Wash the floors, vacuum the rugs, wax the floor, dust your bric-a-brac, scrub pots. Many women, in particular, say that housecleaning lets them work

off nervous tension, besides giving them a sense of accomplishing something. Which you don't get when you stuff your face.

10. Solve puzzles, work crossword puzzles, play word games.

11. Whole-body massage: get one or give one. This strategy combines sensual pleasure with deep relaxation.

12. Play board games like chess, checkers, Monopoly, Scrabble, Clue, backgammon, etc.

13. Go out and look at beautiful scenery. If there's no beautiful scenery in your neighborhood, look at the clouds, at the starry sky, at the raindrops, at the snowflakes, at a rainbow. Look for the beauty in your surroundings. Try to see with a poet's eyes.

14. Shampoo your hair. Enjoy the lather on your scalp and neck. Enjoy the feeling of suds rinsing out of your hair. Then dry your hair very leisurely. Enjoy this as an activity; don't consider taking care of your body to be a chore.

15. Shave. As with shampooing your hair, take time to fully experience the physical sensations of shaving. Learn to enjoy taking care of your body. (This strategy can't be repeated too often, unless you have chronic five-o'clock shadow or are a woman with extremely hairy legs.)

16. Splash your face with cold water, then soak your wrists in cold water. This may be enough of a jolt for some people to stop an impending eating binge.

17. Give or get a manicure. Take your time. Enjoy it. As long as you're clipping and filing and buffing your nails, you can't use those fingers to stuff food down your gullet.

18. Floss your teeth. Use your Water-Pik. Make your mouth feel so fresh and clean that you won't want to defile it with the entry of food.

19. Play trivia games with your friends or quiz yourself on trivia. Examples: Who was Groucho Marx's announcer on the old "You Bet Your Life" television show? List all the actors who've played Tarzan and Superman on TV and in the movies. Give the names of all the actors in the original

206

cast of "Leave It to Beaver." The idea is to get yourself so absorbed in ferreting out obscure facts that you'll forget your urge to overeat.

20. Practice the occult arts—numerology, astrology, tarot.

21. Let somebody else practice the occult arts on you. Have your palm read. Visit a psychic or astrologer for a reading. Visit a gypsy fortuneteller. Concentrate on the future, instead of the present desire to binge. Have fun with these new experiences.

22. Go to a carnival or amusement park. If you ride on the merry-go-round or the roller coaster enough times, you'll get so nauseous that overeating will be the *last* thing on your mind.

23. Go to the zoo. Do *not* feed the animals! Observe how ridiculous the animals look eating the snacks other zoo-goers throw them. You're not an animal; you're a human being, so you don't have to eat whatever's thrown your way. Think how wonderful it is not to be locked up in a cage. But also take time to appreciate the natural beauty of the animals, from the birds' plumage to the glossy coats of the carnivores.

24. Tune in a radio talk show. Phone in and talk to the program's host. Air your views. Feel important—you're on the radio. (Incidentally, this works only if the anxiety of speaking on the radio doesn't cause you to gobble an eclair while on hold before speaking your piece on the airwaves.)

25. Get a job in a bakery, candy store, or ice-cream parlor. You might just OD on your weakness for pastries, sweets, or sundaes and cure your overeating habits. On the other hand, you might just eat yourself into elephantine proportions. Caution: This strategy isn't for everyone.

26. Experiment with a new hair style or a new makeup look. You deserve to look even better than you do now.

27. Write your will. You'll be surprised at how much you have and at how many people you love and wish to remember in your will. You may also realize that being

grossly overweight will shorten your life span, very probably—and you don't want that will to go into effect quite so soon. That's a big impetus to conquer an eating binge.

28. Try gardening. You can do it indoors or outside. Dirty hands are noneating hands. (But don't allow yourself to nibble on the rose petals or to chomp on the fruits you've raised.)

29. Take a long, aimless drive in your car. Concentrating on driving can free your mind from anxiety-producing thoughts that will drive you to eat. (But beware: don't drive into any fast-food franchises for a snack.)

30. Take a long, aimless bus or subway ride. On the bus, you can see new parts of your city. On the subway, you can gaze at strangers' faces and marvel at the infinite diversity of humankind.

31. Daydream. Just stare off into space and let your mind float away. Don't feel guilty for "wool-gathering."

32. Draw or sketch. Keep an artist's pad and charcoals, pastels, or pens handy, so that you don't have to go hunting for your equipment when the urge to overeat strikes.

33. Paint. You can do oils or watercolors or daub the living-room wall. Immerse yourself in the colors and in the manner you apply them to your chosen surface. Get pleasure from your visual senses, as well as from your tongue's sense of taste.

34. Sculpt. Try doing a piece in clay, wood, or even stone. Develop your tactile and spatial senses. Learn to see your art and your surroundings in a new way, a way that deemphasizes the compulsive need to overeat.

35. Wood carving and whittling. This is a highly portable hobby and another good way to increase your awareness and appreciation of your tactile and spatial senses.

36. Make jewelry. And don't just make jewelry for other people. Give yourself a gift of your own jewelry, too.

37. Make pottery. Throwing pots and glazing them is an absorbing activity. The whirling of the potter's wheel is extraordinarily calming, and the work itself is totally absorbing.

38. Make or refinish furniture.

39. Collect antiques, crafts, or art works.

40. Go window shopping in the most elegant part of town or in a large shopping mall that you seldom frequent. Just steer clear, however, of restaurants and gourmet food shops that might lie in your window-shopping path.

41. Go fishing. This is an extremely relaxing pastime (if you angle off a pier) or a challenging one (if you fly-cast while standing in a rushing river, wearing hip boots). It's not how many fish you catch that matters; it's the enjoyment you get from the activity and experience of fishing itself.

42. Engage in an aquatic sport: swimming, diving, snorkeling, scuba diving.

43. Build a fire (in your own fireplace or out in the woods). Then stare into the fire and unwind. This is a very relaxing and sensual experience when fully savored—both primal and transcendent.

44. Go to a movie. It's fine if you go by yourself, in order to stave off an eating binge. Just don't treat yourself to buttered popcorn!

45. Go to a play or a lecture or a poetry reading. Just concentrate wholeheartedly on something other than food for a couple of hours. By then, the urge to binge should have passed.

46. Take a steam bath or a sauna, or sit in one of those outdoor hot tubs so popular on the west coast. Or else just take a plain long soak in your bathtub, with or without bath oil or bubble bath. Enjoy the experience of warm water or air caressing your body. Let your muscle tensions ooze out.

47. Practice yoga. Hatha yoga involves stretching and exercises. Raja yoga focuses more on mental processes and meditation. Both are excellent means of relaxing and of finding a higher meaning in life than stuffing your face.

48. Meditate. Practice Transcendental Meditation or any other form of meditation that you find satisfying and relaxing.

49. Go to a church or synagogue and pray. You don't necessarily have to go to a mass or service. Going alone at

odd hours and sitting and praying can be a more personally meaningful experience than ordinary churchgoing.

50. Drink. Not alcohol (which is both fattening and addictive) but tea, coffee, no-calorie soft drinks, mineral waters, ice water. Give your stomach the illusion of fullness with liquids that don't put on pounds.

51. Repair your car or your spouse's car or your friend's car. Get grease all over your hands. Remember: dirty hands are noneating hands.

52. Take a course in Silva Mind Control and practice its Dynamic Meditation techniques. The Silva course aims at controlling your own mind, not other people's. Silva Mind Control even features special training in methods that help in losing weight and breaking undesirable habits, such as smoking.

53. Practice positive thinking. Repeatedly tell yourself positive messages: "I *will* get thin! I *can* lose weight! I will keep pounds *off!*" Think positively and you'll boost your chances for success.

54. Take training in biofeedback, then practice what you have learned in mind-over-body control at home. Biofeedback is useful not just for weight control but for the feelings of self-mastery it gives you. Increased self-esteem is one notable byproduct.

55. Go to an art gallery or museum. Relish the beauty and drama of colors and forms. Feast your eyes, not your mouth.

56. Go to a library, bookstore, or well-stocked newsstand. Browse and get lost in the reading matter.

57. Chop wood. You can get out your anger and work off some calories, too. Besides, afterward your arms will probably be too stiff and weary to even lift a morsel of food to your mouth.

58. Build models, such as model airplanes or miniature houses or architectural models.

59. Get your desk or bankbook or closet or bookshelves *organized*.

60. Go horseback riding. For the sheer exhilaration of the gallop, for the companionability of the trot.

61. Jog or do long-distance running. Get the legendary runner's high if you can.

62. Try a relatively solitary sport, such as gymnastics, skiing, or a brisk workout in a gym.

63. Try a one-on-one competitive sport, such as tennis, racquetball, handball, squash, or golf. The emphasis shouldn't be on winning but on *involvement*. Throw yourself into the activity. Get pleasure from using your body. And thus, for a little while at least, you just might forget about food.

64. Try a team sport, such as volleyball, baseball, football, basketball, or softball. Again, the emphasis should be on involvement, on enjoying the game for its own sake. A side benefit of team sports is the fact that friendships can be begun and cemented. A drawback of using team sports as an anti-eating strategy is that very often you can't wait long enough to get a team together before you involuntarily embark on an eating binge.

65. Take a long, leisurely walk, preferably in a relaxing environment such as woods, park, or farmland. Or you can watch the cityscape on your walk.

66. Take a course in night school if you tend to overeat most often after dinner. You certainly won't be able to eat while you're in a lecture hall, and you'll have removed yourself, at least temporarily, from the scene of your most trying temptations—home.

67. Play cards. Solitaire, Old Maid, contract bridge, strip poker, or Go Fish—the specific card game doesn't matter. What does matter is that you get involved and interested—and take your mind off food.

68. Read. Novels and histories, in particular, will draw you into another reality—an absorbing, food-free reality. Getting really involved in a long book can fill the empty hours at home when you would ordinarily be hunting desperately for something satisfying to eat.

69. Watch television. (But use this as an anti-eating

strategy only if it's *not* your pattern to eat in front of the TV set.)

70. Take a bicycle ride.

71. Spend the weekend in an isolated cabin, stocked with only nonbinge items and preferably located far from any food stores. This is only for the strong of heart and very determined.

72. To have company or not to have company? If you tend to overeat when you're alone, get company to help cut down on your overeating. Conversely, if you're a social overeater, stay away from parties, and you may diminish your overeating.

73. Throw a party. The planning, cleaning, and preparing will take so much time and energy that you won't think of food.

74. Listen to records or tapes. Close your eyes. Concentrate completely on hearing the music, experiencing the music. Get lost in the waves of sounds.

75. Dance. You can dance around your living room or in a disco or in a ballet or modern-dance class. Get in touch with your body.

76. Take up photography. Then you can wander around town, looking for apt subjects for your lens. Learn to develop your own photos and to print them. Time spent in a darkroom with developing fluid all over your hands is time when you won't eat.

77. Learn a new language. You can do this via records, classes, or phrasebooks with phonetic spelling. In learning a new language, you use your mouth a lot, and that gives you lots of oral compensation for not eating. The newness of the language will require concentration, further distracting you from the thought of food.

78. Work longer hours at your job. (But don't try this anti-eating strategy if you're the workaholic type who eats massive quantities of food after putting in a long day at work.)

79. Take up needlework and knitting. Crewel, needle-

point, bargello, lace-tatting, and crocheting will all keep your hands busy. And busy hands are noneating hands.

80. Walk the dog.

81. Bathe the dog, the cat, the kids.

82. Do dressmaking or tailoring.

83. Try leatherwork.

84. Go to a concert. It doesn't matter if the artist is Vladimir Horowitz or Led Zeppelin. The important thing is that you're partaking of a relaxing and transcendent experience through the music.

85. Go on a religious retreat for the weekend. (But do this only if asceticism doesn't set you off on a backlash binge.)

86. Write a letter—to a friend, to a magazine or newspaper, to a politician, to the manufacturer of an especially good or bad product. It's not the quality of the writing in the letter that matters. The reason for writing the letter is to show yourself that you have significant ideas and opinions and that your opinions matter.

87. Go to a store and try on lots of clothes, both in your current size and in the size you'd like to be if only you could lose the weight. This will give you an incentive to diet, in order to fit into the smaller clothes. It's particularly effective if done regularly, perhaps once a week.

88. Take a directed daydream. Relax yourself completely via meditation or any other technique that works for you. Then close your eyes and imagine that you are at your ideal, fantasized place of relaxation. Voilà—an instant free vacation.

89. Have a controlled food fantasy. This is another form of directed daydream. But this time, instead of going to your ideal place of relaxation in your mind, you're going to eat—but only in your mind. In this daydream, you may consume huge quantities of your favorite fattening foods. You can wallow in these foods; you can mentally swim in lakes of chocolate malts or ski down ice-cream slopes. You can gorge yourself to your heart's content, but you won't

gain an ounce, because all this occurs in your head. It's crucial, however, to continue with the food fantasy until you are completely satiated. Otherwise, the food fantasy might just pique your appetite and set you off on a real binge.

90. Enjoy a good sexual fantasy. Forget your inhibitions. Remember that you are a sexual being, not just an eating one.

91. Make love. As the dieter's proverb goes: Reach for your mate, instead of your plate.

92. Hook a rug.

93. Practice the Relaxation Response. This is a meditation technique that is similar to Transcendental Meditation, but instead of a mantra, you use the word *one* repeatedly to relax.

94. Go to a department store and try on different scents of perfume, cologne, eau de toilette. With practice, you can fit eight or so scents onto your hands and forearms. The scents from department store testers (at the perfume and cosmetic counters) don't cost a cent or a calorie. And they'll open up a new area of sensual pleasure for you—the sense of smell, instead of the sense of taste.

95. Go sailing or motorboating.

96. Take a sightseeing tour in your own city. Act like a tourist for a couple of hours or for the whole day. Guided tours can open up new and interesting areas of your city that you might not have known existed.

97. Sunbathe. Feel the sun on your body. Enjoy it. Bask.

98. Go out and buy a gift for someone you love. Or go out and buy a gift for yourself, because you *deserve* nice things.

99. Go to sleep; take a nap. When you wake up, the urge to binge will probably be gone.

100. Join a club and attend meetings. Get on a committee. By meeting new people and engaging in group activities, you'll have less time to sit at home and eat compulsively.

101. Do volunteer work at a hospital, adult literacy program, social service agency, political campaign, or church. Fill otherwise empty hours with activities and new interests, not with food.

102. Something around your house is probably broken. For once, stop procrastinating, and fix it. Making home improvements and home repairs can stop eating binges.

103. Spend an afternoon or an evening getting to know your body. Bathe, massage yourself, examine. Appreciate how well your body functions. Learn to genuinely like your body because it works. Its shape is less important than its functionality and its uniqueness (its "you-ness").

104. Become your own dental hygienist. Brush your teeth. Gargle with a good-tasting mouthwash. Use one of those plaque-locating tablets that stain plaque reddish pink. If you use a plaque-locating tablet every time you eat, you'll become more aware of how eating dirties up your teeth. You will also spend so much time brushing the tablet's reddish-pink stain off your bicuspids that you simply won't have time to eat.

105. Go out of the house (where food temptation lurks) and do your errands. Do any errands, *except* buying food.

106. Look at your high-school or college yearbook. Reminisce. Remember how good you looked then, and think of how nice it would be to look that way again. (This anti-food strategy isn't right for you if it makes you guilty or melancholy—or if you were fat in high school.)

107. Buy a book of jokes and anecdotes and learn to tell them. This will amuse you and your friends and also help build your self-confidence—you'll never be at a loss for words. (But this strategy, too, has its drawbacks. It's not good to use this if you'll end up turning yourself into the stereotypical jolly fat man/woman.)

108. Recite the names of all fifty states and their capitals before allowing yourself to eat. No cheating! It takes time to do the research on the states and their capitals, and that may provide you with the delay that aborts your eating

binge. Or at least it'll postpone the eating binge, so that you may decrease your voracity.

109. Chew and spit. If you must put some food in your mouth or taste a superfattening delicacy, use this as a last resort. Taste the food, savor it and roll it around your mouth, even chew. But don't swallow. Don't vomit either. Just chew the morsel and spit it out. This is a disgusting strategy, but it works for some people. However, it requires an iron will not to swallow the desired food after chewing.

110. Get involved in a community drama group, either onstage or behind the scenes. Community theater can provide you with camaraderie, involvement, and pride in the eventual production.

111. Get to know your children as people. Talk to them and—more important—listen to them.

112. Relive a romantic moment or incident with your mate. By re-creating this mentally, you may provide yourself with enough remembered satisfaction to overcome today's frustrations and thus avoid a food attack.

113. Make a conscious effort to see with "new" eyes. That is, look for the beautiful and the bizarre in your daily environment. Stop taking your surroundings for granted, and you may be surprised at the wealth of new and fascinating things you discover.

114. Count your blessings.

115. Have your blood pressure taken or get the equipment to test it yourself and learn how to conduct this procedure. This may be especially effective if you require a health incentive to lose weight. If you lose weight, high blood pressure symptoms very often will abate. Lowering your blood pressure should be a compelling reason not to binge. However, you shouldn't weigh yourself too. That's one of the best ways to initiate a cycle of guilt, self-deprivation, and binge. And you don't need *that*.

116. Treat yourself to some "luxury" that you previously denied yourself because you weren't thin enough or because you had broken your diet. The luxury treat may be an article

of clothing or theater tickets or a book or a status symbol/ nonessential. The point isn't to spend a fortune. The point is to show yourself that you can be good to yourself without resorting to food.

117. Take out your anger on a certain person (the one who is "driving" you to eat) by holding an imaginary conversation with that person. If your boss or your mate is getting you so edgy that you want to overeat, tell that person off. But do it in an imaginary conversation if actually telling the person off would cause serious harm—such as losing your job or your spouse.

118. Expel the anger and aggression that are triggering an overeating binge by attacking a punching bag or by beating rugs or just by pummeling a pillow. Express your hostility before you turn it inward and wind up with self-hate, which leads to overeating.

119. Plan a trip to an exotic or exciting locale. Visit travel agents and government tourist offices. Collect brochures and maps. Learn all you can about this desired vacation spot. Then take a trip in your fantasies as an escape.

120. With your eyes closed, fantasize about how wonderful you'll feel and look once you've reached your desired weight. Fantasize about how people will react to you when you're slimmer. Visualize yourself at your ideal weight—feel it, enjoy it. Now it won't seem so impossible to reach your goal and to stay there. In this way, you can reprogram your mind to think like a thin person, instead of thinking like an overweight person.

121. Turn out the lights. If you must eat, make yourself do it in the dark. Oddly enough, eating in the dark completely turns off most people's appetites—probably because food is desirable only as long as you can see it. This cuts down on your electricity bills, too.

If none of these 121 strategies works for you, sit down and think of some of the most relaxing and pleasurable things you like to do—the things you'd like to do but usually don't, for one reason or another. Make a list of those things. Tape a copy on the refrigerator door. Keep another copy of the list in your wallet. These are your alternatives.

Look at your alternatives *before* you start your overeating. As long as you're aware that you have many alternatives to food, you have a better chance of controlling your compulsive eating.

The whole key to finding alternatives to overeating is summed up in this phrase: *expand your repertoire of behavior.*

Most overeaters keep turning to food because it's a habit, because other, nonfattening alternatives don't immediately come to mind. With your list of anti-eating strategies that work for you, you do have alternatives. You do have things you can do—other than feeding your face.

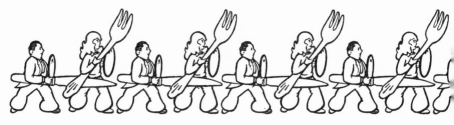

# 14   The Realistic Body

All right, you've tried the alternatives to eating and over-eating. You've gotten involved in community affairs. You've made sure you don't eat alone or late at night or at a party—whichever situation is your particular undoing. You've stopped eating in the car, in your bedroom, in front of the TV, standing up in front of the refrigerator. You've done crossword puzzles, needlepoint, and carpentry to keep your hands too busy to stuff your face full of calories.

And what happens? You *still* don't like the way you look. Your body is "wrong." The thighs are too pudgy. Or you've still got a (slightly deflated) spare tire around the mid-section. Or your backside is still swaying way out behind you like some sort of fleshy caboose.

You've tried everything, and you still don't look the way you want to. You still don't look thin *enough*.

Now you have to consider the fact that you may have an unrealistic idea of what your own body could or should look like. Most people in this thin-obsessed society have unrealistic ideas of the proper body shape and size.

In the chapter called "Culture 'Talks' Thin," you got some idea of how brainwashed members of this society are about thinness. Slimness is considered the key to sex appeal, business success, health, youthfulness, and a plethora of other positive goals. Our culture grants thinness *magical* attributes, as if being slender, in and of itself, could solve virtually all our problems.

As a result of our cultural conditioning, most of us want to be not just "average" weight but thin, extremely thin. For women, the goal is to be fashion-model slim. For men, the super-leanness of track stars is an ideal. Thinness is just part of these body-shape goals. The body proportions this culture celebrates are long, angular, leggy, flat-stomached, high-breasted, and firm-bottomed.

But for most people, these idealized body shapes are simply not realistic. By adopting these goals for yourself, you may be engaging in an ultimately self-defeating, self-destructive activity. Often people in their rapt Pursuit of Thin do not take into account the basic, built-in shape of their bodies—a shape dictated by genetic, metabolic, and structural factors that are largely beyond our control.

Even after arduous food deprivation and attaining the "proper" weight for their height, many women still have disproportionately heavy thighs, and some men still have a disproportionate midsection bulge. These are simply the ways in which their bodies are innately programmed to distribute fat and muscle tissues. Thus, their body shapes and forms derive more from centuries of genetic heritage than from a bout on the latest wonder diet.

Animals come in varied breeds, and so do people. For instance, Aberdeen Angus cattle fatten up faster than other breeds of cattle—and they're prized for this attribute. In the canine world, dogs may be judged "best in show" whether they're roly-poly Old English sheepdogs, elegantly lanky Afghan hounds, or petite Yorkshire terriers. Just as animal breeds differ in appearance and in the way in which they put on fat, people also differ in their possible ideal shapes and in the ways they gain or lose weight.

Perhaps you may be better able to visualize this concept by considering various ethnic groups as very loosely defined "breeds" of sorts. Certainly, most people from southern

Italy look different from most people whose ethnic heritage stems from northern Scandinavia or from equatorial Africa. This can be proved by the fact that there are measurable ethnic differences in obesity in the United States population.

In his 1936 studies, published as *What Is an American?*, the physical anthropologist Earnest A. Hooton showed that the "least obese" Americans are those who come from Scottish, Irish, and "old American" stock (families who have lived in the United States for many generations). A slightly more obesity-prone group of Americans, according to Hooton's data, are those of German or Scandinavian background. And the most obese group of Americans, Hooton's studies found, are persons of Eastern European descent, specifically Central Slavs, Soviet Russians, and Balto-Ugrics (people from Latvia, Estonia, and Lithuania).

Further Hooton studies have shown that people in some areas of the United States tend to be thinner as a group than people in other geographical regions, whatever their ethnic backgrounds. People from the southeastern states are found to be the leanest, while the fattest Americans tend to come from the mid-Atlantic and midwestern regions.

Why should these ethnic and geographical differences in levels of obesity occur? Climate is one possible factor. People from warmer climates may have less need for body fat to keep them warm in winter months. Also, they may engage in more year-round outdoor physical activities because of the opportunities offered by warm climates. Warm weather allows these people to wear fewer clothes, too, and so they're more conscious of the shape of their bodies and of their general physical condition than people from colder climates, where bodies are shrouded in layers of heavy clothing for a good part of the year.

As to ethnic variances in obesity levels, climatic factors may once again come into play. Ethnic variances in obesity may also be accounted for by differences in ethnic cooking, eating, emphasis on food as a social force, and concepts of ideal body weight and shape. These ethnic cultural messages may help to shape our bodies in many subtle ways.

Intriguingly, it may not be how much you eat but how your body uses food that determines your weight. The same number of calories puts different amounts of weight on different people. These differences in weight gain are attributed to inherent metabolic factors—not to sloth, lack of self-discipline, or psychopathology.

Depending on an individual's metabolism, only 1,200 calories may add a pound of fat onto his body, or as many as 3,500 calories may be needed to add that pound of fat. European scientists have long discussed this phenomenon as relating to "the caloric cost of the kilo" (one kilo equals 2.2 pounds). Thus, scientist M. J. Demole wrote that, depending on a given person's genetic-metabolic constitution, he can need anywhere from 6,000 calories down to 2,500 calories to gain a kilo.

If a person requires 6,000 surplus calories to gain 2.2 pounds, he naturally tends to stay thinner than an "easy gainer." The obesity-prone individual possesses the "thrifty gene." His body naturally tends to expend energy slowly and to retain calories easily in the form of fat. People with thrifty genes tend to conserve calories—and fat. Thus, this type of person might be able to put on 2.2 pounds by ingesting just 2,500 extra calories.

And so, even on identical diets—consuming the same number and same type of calories—some people will lose weight, but other people with "thrifty genes" may actually gain weight. The key to whether you gain or lose weight is the manner in which your body metabolizes food (fuel in the form of calories).

This brings up a thorny question. Do you get fat because you eat too much? Or do you eat too much because you're genetically *programmed* to run to fat?

Recently, physical anthropologists have put forth an intriguing new theory of obesity. They hypothesize that people who put on weight easily (i.e., people who tend to have a weight problem) may, in fact, be responding to urges and metabolic processes that are genetically built into them. The woman who can't squeeze into a size 18 dress and the man who bursts the seams of a size 44 jacket may not be undisciplined gluttons after all. Instead, physical anthropologists theorize that these fleshier people may look as they do and may weigh as much as they do because of events that occurred thirty thousand years ago!

These social scientists think that during the last Ice Age, it was a survival trait to use calories slowly and sparingly— the very factors that today create the bane of overweight. In those Ice Age (Paleolithic) times, the food supply was sparse and erratic, dependent largely on luck in hunting. A Paleolithic man or woman who was "calorically frugal" (who used up food calories slowly) would have a better chance of surviving in that bitter and brutal climate, when European winters might last for ten months of the year.

The calorically thrifty individuals of that period could bounce back more easily from the repeated pattern of feast (the hunters have come home with a big kill) and famine (the hunters have come home empty-handed). By using their calories slowly, these calorically thrifty people maximized their chances for survival. They were better able to endure the famine periods since their bodies released calories (stored in fat tissues) more slowly. This trait enabled these Paleolithic ancestors of ours to live through that extra day, week, or month when food was scarce or nonexistent. They endured famine and deprivation and lived to pass those calorically thrifty genetic patterns on to their offspring.

And thirty thousand years after the last Ice Age, the physical anthropologists suggest that the descendants of these hardy Paleolithic survivors became precisely the fleshy, fat-prone people who end up patronizing fat farms and amphetamine-happy diet doctors. Instead of being proud of their survival factor, today's calorically thrifty people feel doomed to a lifetime of fighting the battle of the bulge.

The physical anthropologists offer another theory why so

many middle-aged people put on weight. It's a fact that middle-aged and elderly people will gain weight if they continue to eat the same number of calories as they did when they were younger. The inactivity of their increasingly sedentary lives might be one causal factor. Or their bodies might be effortlessly, instinctively turning more calories into fat tissues.

This, too, might be the result of another prehistoric survival trait that has been genetically programmed into some people. In these more primitive times, older people may have been less able to hunt and gather foods. Since they were less able than younger people to obtain large quantities of food (calories), the older people's bodies became calorically thriftier with age. Making do with fewer calories enhanced the older person's chances for survival. Today, however, we don't thank this survival factor in our genetic heritage—we blame it for creating middle-aged spread.

## ARE BINGES GENETICALLY PROGRAMMED?

We can even speculate that the diet-binge pattern that many compulsive eaters experience has some underlying genetic reasons. The binge period is a feast, and the diet period is a self-imposed famine. Thus, modern-day men and women are unwittingly re-creating the eating patterns of ancestors who died more than three hundred centuries ago: feast and famine, binge and diet. Perhaps the overwhelming desire to binge has some grounds not just in social, cultural, and psychological factors but also in our innate genetic programming, the legacy of ancient mankind.

## FAT BABIES, FAT CELLS, FAT ADULTS

Of course, you don't have to go back to Paleolithic times to find reasons why you look more like Henry VIII than Mark Spitz, more like Totie Fields than Twiggy. The physiological reasons for your size and shape may have occurred months before you were even born. You may have been doomed to pudginess or skinniness in your mother's womb.

224

A study by Dr. Mervyn W. Susser and Dr. Zena A. Stein of the Columbia University School of Public Health supports just that conclusion. Susser and Stein based their study on the weights of almost ninety-five thousand men who were born in the Netherlands during a World War II famine. The study showed that men whose mothers suffered a food shortage during the first six months of pregnancy tended to be overweight. However, a baby who (because of this wartime famine) was poorly nourished during the last three months in the womb and during the first few months of life tended to become a skinny adult.

Similarly, findings by Dr. Fredda Ginzberg of New York's Mount Sinai Hospital School of Medicine show that a sweet tooth can be developed long before the infant has its first tooth erupt from its gums. "Even a fetus in the uterus can develop a sweet tooth from its mother's diet during the last three months of pregnancy," Dr. Ginzberg reported.

American baby formulas are high in sugar content, and these "very sweet formulas" fed to a baby in infancy may inadvertently develop a sweet tooth in the baby that persists into adulthood, according to Dr. Ginzberg.

An infant with an excessive appetite usually turns into a child and an adult with an excessive appetite. One reason for this very hungry infant might be that the child is born with too much insulin in its bloodstream. Insulin is known to increase hunger, so the baby is naturally more hungry than average. An elevated infant insulin level is also sometimes associated with infants whose mothers were diabetic during pregnancy.

Prenatal factors also tie into the "fat cell" theory of overweight. Recent studies demonstrate that if a mother is obese during her pregnancy, she may bear a child who has a higher percentage of fat cells than average.

What do fat cells have to do with overweight? According to many physiologists, excessive fat cells doom a person to overweight—or, at the very least, to having to maintain constant vigilance against overweight. Surplus calories are stored in the body in fat tissues. These fat tissues are composed of many fat cells. After age ten to fifteen, the number of fat cells that each person has remains constant during the rest of his or her lifetime.

When a person is at her heaviest weight, her fat cells are also fat—they are full. When such a person loses weight, the fat cells don't disappear or decrease in number. Instead, these cells empty part of their contents and become smaller, thinner. According to Dr. Marci Greenwood of the Institute of Human Nutrition, obesity-prone people may have up to five times more fat cells than average.

Women generally have many more fat cells than men, which makes women as a group more prone to overweight and more resistant to losing weight. Women and men distribute their fat cells and, hence, fat tissues differently, too. Men typically accumulate their fat ventrally (around the abdomen). However, women typically accumulate their fat dorsally (around the back of the body). This accounts for why men tend to put weight on first in the form of paunches, while women are more prone to concentrate their overweight in the hips and derriere.

With very few exceptions, all overweight people have enlarged fat cells. When dieting decreases the size of these fat cells, an undesirable side effect may occur in these "naturally obese" individuals: the depleted fat cells send urgent messages to the brain and appetite centers. These messages are the fat cells' SOS—"Send more food, we're starving." This may create a tremendous, irrational urge to eat in those fat-prone individuals who have many more fat cells than average.

Another gloomy fact about fat cells: most of them are formed either before birth or in the first few months or years of life. Thus, a cute, chubby baby is crawling around with a time bomb inside his body—an excessive number of fat cells. And so the chubby baby will turn into a plump schoolchild and then into an obese adolescent and adult. In a very real sense, this person isn't completely to blame for his overweight—his overabundant fat cells make losing weight and maintaining that weight loss very, very difficult.

Between 12 and 16 percent of American children and adolescents are judged obese. This isn't just "baby fat" which disappears when a kid turns sweet sixteen or goes off to college. Studies indicate that fully 85 percent of obese children will remain fat into adulthood.

## FAMILIES AND OVERWEIGHT

Overweight also seems to run in families. A child with two obese parents has an 80 percent chance of being obese. A child with only one obese parent has a 40 percent chance of being obese. A child with two parents of average weight, however, has only a 10 percent chance of growing up overweight or obese.

A survey of eating habits and nutritional status of a large representative group of Americans turned up more distressing statistics about fat running in families. On the whole, the children of obese parents were found, in this survey, to be heavier than the children of thin or average-weight parents. By the time the children of obese parents turned seventeen, they were actually three times fatter than the children of thin parents. And, according to the survey, these overweight children of the obese continued to gain weight until the end of their teenage years, making their weight problems even more acute.

Why does overweight run in families? One explanation postulates that overweight is largely determined by heredity, metabolic patterns with genetic programming as their basis. Another explanation holds that the children of obese parents are conditioned in childhood to overeat, because their parents overfeed them and encourage them to overeat. In this way, these children may form a lifelong habit of overeating.

Both explanations are persuasive, and any complete understanding of overweight cannot exclude either set of factors—the hereditary and the environmental. It's the old nature versus nurture debate, translated into the terms of obesity.

## DIFFERENT SHAPES FOR DIFFERENT FOLKS

Fat may run in your family or in your ethnic group or in your region of the United States. Fat may be programmed into you because you were overfed as a baby and developed too many fat cells or because you were born with too much insulin in your bloodstream and developed a voracious appetite—and a lot of fat cells. Fat may be genetically programmed into you because you are descended from hardy, fat-prone people who survived the last Ice Age. There are untold reasons why you tend to be fat, why you aren't thin or thin enough.

Have you ever considered the idea that maybe you *shouldn't* be thin? Maybe your basic body build fights against being thin, just as much as your overtaxed willpower fights against the temptation of a gooey hot-fudge sundae.

Earlier, it was briefly mentioned that various breeds of dogs may look widely different yet still be perfect—*for their type.* A champion show dog doesn't have to be a slender greyhound or whippet. It can be a burly Saint Bernard or a middleweight fox terrier. No one breed or shape of dog is considered the *only* right shape.

Why should we think that only one shape of man or woman is the "right" shape? The current style may be to look like John Travolta or Cheryl Tiegs, like Robert Redford or Farrah Fawcett. And because these people's body shapes are now in style, most of us assume that this is the *only* way to look, the only way to be built. Nothing could be further from the truth.

People come in all sizes and shapes, and no one shape is really more normal or more perfect or more innately desirable than another.

A good example of the multiplicity of perfectly functioning body types can be seen every four years at the Olympics. Different sports demand different body shapes. Female gymnasts must be fairly short, slender, and extremely flexible. And so we see Olympic competitors who look like Nadia Comaneci or Olga Korbut. Weight lifters, on the other hand, must be muscle-packed, with much of their weight and strength concentrated in the midsection to achieve maximum "lift." And so we see bodies like that of the Soviet superheavyweight gold medalist Vasili Alexeev. Alexeev weighs about three hundred imposing pounds, with not only monumental shoulder, arm, and thigh muscles but also a vastly protruding, all-muscle pot belly—the better to lift weights with.

Alexeev and Comaneci are both gold medalists—the best in the world at what they do physically. And certainly any Olympic champion must be in superlative physical condition. But Comaneci is elfin, petite, and Alexeev is gargantuan, hulking. This just goes to prove that no one body type or body shape is "right." Comaneci made her body the best of its type (the human equivalent of the dog show's "best of breed"). But that doesn't mean that the only right body type is that of a world-class female gymnast.

Human bodies come in a pleasing, albeit puzzling, array of shapes and sizes. And no one has analyzed, photographed, and recorded this splendid diversity more comprehensively than William Herbert Sheldon. Sheldon was the first to fully develop and document the manifold possibilities of human body builds. He called his body builds "somatotypes."

In his influential book on body types, published in 1940, Sheldon coined three words to denote the basic types of physiques. The first of these somatotypes was the endomorphic. A typical endomorph would be light-boned, fleshy, and well-padded. At the opposite extreme of body types from the endomorphic in Sheldon's system is the ectomorphic. A typical ectomorph would be skeletally fragile, long-legged, and linear or angular. Between the endomorphs and the ectomorphs stand the mesomorphs. The mesomorphic characteristics imply that this person would be skeletally sturdy, muscular, and broad-shouldered.

Let's bring Sheldon's system down to specifics. A complete endomorph might look like King Henry VIII (in his famous Holbein portrait done during his corpulent middle age) or like the rotund English actor Robert Morley or like the TV show "Hee Haw's" country-singing dumpling Lulu Roman. A complete mesomorph might look like Olympic swimming star Mark Spitz or marathon swimmer Diana Nyad or football quarterback Joe Namath or soccer great Pelé. The complete ectomorph might be represented by fashion models such as Twiggy or Cheryl Tiegs or by film stars such as the young Katharine Hepburn, Audrey Hepburn, Henry Fonda, and Jimmy Stewart.

Of course, almost no one is purely endomorphic, ectomorphic, or mesomorphic. Sheldon believed—and his research supported the supposition—that people are a mixture of all these traits, though one of these somatotypes predominates in each person.

Sheldon and his associates classified people on a 1-to-7 scale in each of the three main somatotypes. A 1 score in endomorphic characteristics might mean a person had very little fat on him, but he might score a 5 in mesomorphic traits and a 4 in ectomorphic traits. Thus, this person would tend to be slim but muscular. A ballet dancer might have such a somatotype. But a football fullback might score a 6 in mesomorphic traits, a 5 in endomorphy, and a 2 in ectomorphy. Both the ballet dancer and the fullback may have "beautiful" bodies. But they're very different kinds of beauty.

Sheldon's research has larger implications than just being able to classify people's body builds scientifically on a worldwide basis. And his research is more than just another parlor game whereby you and your friends try to classify acquaintances on a scale of 1 to 7 for endomorphy, ectomorphy, and mesomorphy.

The real message of Sheldon's research is that people come in all sorts of sizes and shapes. And since we each start out with a unique body type, it's fruitless to try to reshape that body into the current limited concept of what is normal, what is beautiful, what is sexy.

Yet one of the most irritating and painful teachings in our culture and media is that only a few, a very few of these numerous body types can be considered "ideal." Using the categories Sheldon developed, there are eighty-eight body types among Caucasian males. But only about three of these body types—men whom Sheldon referred to as "extreme mesomorphs"—are considered "ideal" by our culture and media. These extreme mesomorphs are muscular with large shoulders, slim hips, and narrow waists.

If a man is one of the other eighty-five body types, he's out of luck. What usually happens is that he spends half his life trying to make himself look like the extreme mesomorph he was never born to be. If he's naturally of ectomorphic build, he'll try to build muscles, attacking those barbells and Nautilus weight machines with vigor—and a little desperation. If he tends toward fleshy endomorphy, he'll spend his life trying to firm up, utilizing every conceivable method from jogging and steam baths to the latest miracle diet. Since these people aren't innately built in the "ideal" male shape of today, the extreme mesomorph physique, they spend their lives trying to be something they're not ever going to be.

(There is *some* justice here, however. Sheldon found that even "extreme mesomorphs" looked their best only in late adolescence. These body types tend to get thicker in middle age; they gain an average of fifteen pounds, get wider in the waist, and generally lose their granite-muscle contours. So even extreme mesomorphs—those born with the "ideal" body shape—must spend most of their adult years battling to keep trim, to maintain their late-adolescent "perfect" physiques.)

To take it back to canine analogies, no matter how hard an Old English sheepdog diets or runs in the fields, he's not going to turn into a slim greyhound or a sleek Afghan hound. Similarly, a Yorkshire terrier is never going to add enough weight and size to even begin to resemble a golden retriever.

Just as a dog cannot change from one breed to another simply by force of will (and force of diet and exercise), people cannot change from one somatotypic "breed" to another. If you're primarily ectomorphic, you're going to spend a lot of your life drinking Nutrament to gain weight or else parading around in a size 6 dress, glorying in your skinniness.

If you're primarily of the endomorphic "breed," you might as well accept the fact that you can't change your basic body pattern. You can't make yourself leggier or more "skeletally fragile," to use Sheldon's terminology. If you're of the endomorphic breed, you're going to have to fight the battle of the bulge all your life. Because your body knows the shape it was meant to be naturally and tries to keep itself that way, even if you think it's too fat. That endomorphic, rounded, fleshy body may be a great body, a beautifully functioning body. But you might never learn to appreciate it, because your body is not in style.

That's right—style.

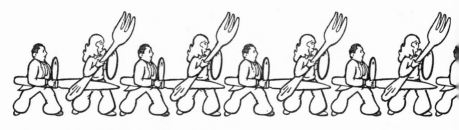

# 15 Body Styles versus Being the Best Possible You

Body shapes come into and go out of style just the way clothes do. Today's "ugly" body may be yesterday's ideal of beauty or handsomeness. A body too fat by contemporary Western standards may be deemed "just right" in other parts of the world. Attitudes toward physical perfection, toward the Body Beautiful, have varied widely in different historical periods.

For most of the past five hundred years, fat has been in style, and thin has been out of fashion. It has been only in the last fifty years or so that slenderness has become the ideal and the obsession of the industrialized Western nations.

Today we associate thinness with looking youthful, but this wasn't always so. The seventeenth-century English poet John Dryden wrote, "I am resolved to grow fat and look young till forty." Clearly, in Dryden's era, plumpness was associated with the bloom of youth, while the gaunt, emaciated look was associated with old age and death. Today the person with that gaunt, emaciated look is on the cover of a fashion magazine, and the plump person is hiding in the bedroom, stuffing Mallomars into her mouth while thinking how embarrassing it is not to be svelte.

In cultures where food is often in short supply, thinness will never be considered beautiful. Instead, slimness will bear connotations of famine and suffering. Perhaps that's why the Hottentots of Africa (who often face severe food shortages) covet women with hugely bulging buttocks and stomachs. The women are grotesquely fat and ill-proportioned to modern Western eyes. But to the Hottentots such women reek of prosperity, of having plenty of food to eat.

Another case of *preferring* fat occurs in the Middle East. Arab men feel girth is manly, a sign of prosperity and even of power. Arabs have also traditionally considered the voluptuous, well-padded female shape far more beautiful than the slender androgyny now favored in the West.

The pre-twentieth-century Hawaiians considered body fat and sheer body mass to signify not only beauty and handsomeness but nobility as well. Fatness showed that a person possessed more *mana,* more power drawn from the divinities. Some of their kings ate their way up to 400 pounds, in order to appear fatter and hence more majestic and divine to their subjects. The Hawaiian queens, too, favored the well-endowed look. A photograph of Queen Kapiolani, taken around 1882, shows a formidable beauty of over 250 solidly packed pounds.

When Christian missionaries came to Hawaii in the nineteenth century, they were aghast to see so much flesh, however majestic, displayed so openly. (The Hawaiians liked bare flesh just as much as sheer volume of flesh itself.) To cover the hefty Hawaiian beauties, the missionaries devised a loose, shapeless gown, called a muumuu, which completely concealed the sinfully tempting, voluptuous flesh of the female islanders.

In present-day Tonga, an island nation in Polynesia, the people are proud of their fatness. There, overweight (by Western standards) is considered the mark of high social standing, as well as of good health. This ideal of fatness as good looks is exemplified in the monumental figure of Tonga's monarch, King Taufa'ahau Tupou IV, who tips the scales at 380 pounds.

The nonroyal Tongans strain to achieve *sino le le,* which means "healthy fullness," in their body shape. A visiting

Englishman in 1902 described the Tongan conception of female beauty this way: "The perfect woman must be fat— that is most imperative—and her neck must be short; she must have no waist . . . ; her bust, hips, and thighs must be colossal. The woman who possesses all these perfections will be esteemed chief-like and elegant. . . ." Today's Tongans still adhere to roughly those ideals of beauty, despite adopting many other forms of Westernization.

Arabs, Hawaiians, Tongans, or Hottentots—this preference for the plump or even fat form is not uncommon around the world. In fact, except in the affluent, industrialized West, most of the Earth's peoples and cultures extol the plump over the slim, especially where women's body builds are concerned.

As one anthropologist reported in the Human Relations Area Files, "As far as general body build is concerned, the majority of societies whose preferences in this matter are recorded feel that a plump woman is more attractive than a thin one."

Other entries in the anthropological Human Relations Area Files stress that heaviness is positively erotic in many cultures. Witness the entry regarding the Sirione people of the Brazilian Amazon River basin: "Besides being young, a desirable sex partner should also be fat. She should have big hips, good-sized but firm breasts, and a deposit of fat on her sexual organs."

But you don't have to journey to Africa, Polynesia, South America, or even the Middle East to find examples of fat being in style. Just go back into the past of European and North American culture, and you can find numerous examples. In fact, it might well be said that beauty is in the *era* of the beholder.

The earliest known European sex symbol wasn't slender. She was, by today's Western standards, horribly fat. This "sex symbol" is the Paleolithic sculpture called the Venus of Willendorf, a rotund, nude figurine with a globular stomach, bulging hips and buttocks, pendulous breasts, and thick thighs. Certainly not a candidate for Miss America.

Art historians estimate that if this stout, 4⅜-inch sculpture were elongated to today's average female heights, the Venus of Willendorf would boast measurements of 96–89–96 inches. Not a beauty by today's standards at all. But to Ice-Age European hunting peoples, such blatantly fat female statuettes represented their sexy ideal.

The ancient Egyptians favored a fairly lean body build, as evidenced by their tomb paintings and statuary. The ancient Greeks and Romans admired taut stomachs and abundant musculature in their men. However, a certain degree of male heaviness connoted maturity and power. The ancient Greeks and Romans did have some strange standards of feminine beauty; the famed Greek sculptor Praxiteles demanded that the perfect female body had to have the navel centered exactly between the breasts and genitals.

Although the ancient Greeks and Romans did not immortalize females with the sheer girth of the Ice-Age Venus of Willendorf, they did favor a more matronly body build than do contemporary Westerners. The statue of the Venus de Milo—generally considered the ancient world's ideal of feminine beauty—is decidedly thick in the waist. And her hips measure a more-than-robust forty-eight inches. Clearly, the ancient Greeks and Romans accepted and even glorified plumpness.

Europe in the Middle Ages had rather ambivalent ideas about what the ideal body—male or female—should look like. Most medieval art shows fairly thin people, sometimes scrawny to the point of angularity. Yet the females are frequently shown with bulging stomachs, probably to signify or to imitate pregnancy; fertility was esteemed then.

Medieval European Christians preached against gluttony. It was, after all, one of the Big Seven—the seven deadly sins, along with such goodies as lust, pride, and avarice. But Europeans of the Middle Ages did admire the "well-fed" look of the nobility and well-to-do townspeople. Most of the medieval peasantry eked out a bare subsistence living. People who had enough money to be heavyset were, therefore, people of financial greatness and often social prominence—the elite.

To the Europeans of the Middle Ages, plumpness equaled prosperity. And prosperity equaled God's grace or favor. Thus, gluttony was abhorred, but plumpness was honored.

Plumpness, though not gluttonous obesity, was also considered attractive in the Renaissance, as attested by the beatific, round-faced Madonnas and noblewomen of Leonardo da Vinci's paintings. Michelangelo's famed statue of David—an extreme mesomorph with broad shoulders, muscled arms and legs, and narrow waist—set a standard of male beauty for centuries. Yet Michelangelo's broad-chested, muscled young man—so much like the current ideal—went out of favor for a couple of hundred years.

In the eighteenth century, the English painter Thomas Gainsborough presented portraits of gentlemen who were actually big-bellied. These men's shoulders were narrow, and they were quite long-waisted and hollow-chested. This was the desired body style of that period.

Eventually, the Gainsborough-pictured masculine idea gave way to a new male body style. In the early 1800s, short waists and long, muscled legs came into vogue. Men wore skintight pantaloons that mercilessly displayed the "good turn" (or lack of it) in the legs. This fashion also called attention to the man's crotch—a prominent genital bulge was *de rigueur,* if a man wanted his body shape to conform to fashion's dictates.

During the Victorian period, the bulging stomach again returned as high style in male bodies. A bulge—often called an embonpoint—was necessary if a gentleman wanted to look prosperous. Cummerbunds and other articles of clothing called attention to the embonpoint. And if a gentleman had, alas, a flat stomach, he often sought to conceal this defect by padding himself around the midriff.

Then, just as suddenly, men found that body styles had dramatically shifted. The military look was in, and that demanded a narrow midsection. According to one 1903

English news report, "The corset mania began with the military men; they compare notes on corsets in some of the army clubs as gravely as they discuss the education bill at the National Library Club."

The well-fed look had a resurgence in the postwar years of the late 1940s and 1950s. But by the 1960s, rock music idols and the counterculture spawned a skinny-is-in image for young men. They dieted and struggled to look hollow-chested in their T-shirts, trying to shrink into reasonable facsimiles of such scrawny rock superstars as Mick Jagger and David Bowie.

Today the male body style has shifted somewhat to the long-distance runner look—superlean but somewhat muscled, nevertheless. Body builders with Herculean builds like Arnold Schwarzenegger are considered rather freakishly overmuscled by today's body styles for men. But fatness is considered even more abhorrent. Virtually the only heavy-set men you'll see on national television are clowns and bigots like Archie Bunker of "All in the Family." Just about everybody else on TV, from newsmen to the Fonz and Mork from Ork, are slim and trim. Because in this era, in this culture, thin is once again in.

If you think men's body styles have changed over the years, you'll be amazed at the different shapes women have tried to mold their bodies into. Until this century, almost all ideals of female beauty in art represented rather hefty women, ranging from pleasantly plump to downright chubby.

For instance, in Titian's *Venus and the Lute Player,* a sublime example of the sixteenth-century Venetian High Renaissance style, Venus's body is a series of soft, almost exploding curves. Even her elbow is barely angular. Titian has defined the body style of his era's women and exemplifies it in his Venus's plump thighs, gently rounded calves and arms, nearly pleated folds of flesh at the stomach. This Venus is heavyset by today's standards. But by the standards of the sixteenth century, Titian's age, this Venus is beauty incarnate. She is her era's ideal of body style.

In seventeenth-century art, consider the women painted by Peter Paul Rubens. In Rubens's *The Three Graces,* three women—enormously fat by today's standards—cavort in the nude. Their hips and buttocks are pillowy. Their thighs are dimpled with fat. Their flesh is luminously pink and abundant, so abundant that the fat becomes opulent and seductive. Today Rubens's Three Graces would be begged by their relatives to commit themselves to some fat farm for a lengthy incarceration, so that they could starve themselves into some semblance of "normal" weight. But in the seventeenth century, Rubens's Three Graces conformed to the reigning body style. And so they were deemed beautiful—the Charlie's Angels of their day.

Female body styles continued to change. In the court of Louis XIV, the French Sun King, the female waist was cinched in, the bosom was flattened, and the hips were made to look enormous with wired and padded undergarments.

Body styles had shifted by the Napoleonic era. Then a neoclassical vogue exposed bodies to greater scrutiny (through skimpier garments made of sheerer materials). Bosoms were supposed suddenly to become small and high, hips and buttocks neatly trim. Waistlines were unimportant, since many dresses were Empire-waisted (tied under the bosom).

By the middle of the nineteenth century, however, the tiny waistline became a necessity, and tightly laced corsets nearly made breathing impossible for many ladies who wanted to conform to the current body style. (Margaret Mitchell recalled those days of cinched-in waist and voluminously hoop-skirted hips in *Gone with the Wind*—remember Scarlett O'Hara's acclaimed eighteen-inch waist?) Rubens and Titian would have thought such unnaturally tiny waistlines sickly, not beautiful.

Later in the nineteenth century, Lillie Langtry popularized the hourglass figure—small waist with the excess midsection flesh seemingly displaced by corsets into the bosom and hips. The hourglass figure resembled an old-style Coca

Cola bottle—but with a smaller midsection. Yet Langtry, the greatest beauty of her day, would have been considered overweight by today's standards—she weighed about 135 pounds, at 5 feet 4 inches.

Lillian Russell, the most famous sex symbol of late nineteenth-century America, had not only a double chin, but billowing hips, thighs, and buttocks, and she easily weighed more than 150 pounds. She and her lover, Diamond Jim Brady, used to entertain themselves by seeing who could eat more—and a lot of Lillian's eating victories went straight to her chunky thighs. Yet men of that period would drool over photographs of Lillian Russell—because she exemplified the luxuriously plump body style of the time.

At the turn of the twentieth century, body styles made another shift, though plumpness was still highly regarded. The Gibson-girl look, epitomized by the illustrations of Charles Dana Gibson, became the fashionable body style. The Gibson girl was noticeably buxom; she had what was termed the "pouter-pigeon bosom." Her stomach was full and pouchy, and she was also supposed to sport a fashionable sway-backed stance. This physical transformation—or distortion, depending on your point of view—was achieved mostly through skillful corseting.

A certain fleshiness was considered essential for feminine beauty even during the early decades of the twentieth century. The turn-of-the-century American beauty expert Harriet Hubbard Ayer wrote that "the hollow-cheeked, angular, flat-chested woman cannot be really physically lovely. . . ." Today such a woman might be a $100-an-hour fashion model.

Mrs. Ayer also included a table of ideal weights in her well-known health and beauty guide. These "proper weights" are far more than what is considered suitable for the body style of today. Mrs. Ayer said a 5-foot-1-inch woman should weigh 120 pounds; a 5-foot-2-inch woman should weigh 126 pounds; and a 5-foot-10-inch "giantess" should weigh at least 174 pounds.

Compare this to today's ideals. Fashion model Cheryl

Tiegs is 5 feet 10½ inches tall. Her "working weight" for photographic and television modeling is no more than 120 pounds. But at her fattest (and most unemployable as a model), Tiegs said she once "ballooned to 150 pounds." By turn-of-the-century standards, Tiegs wouldn't be a paragon of beauty. Instead, she'd be considered unattractively scrawny—and about 50 pounds *underweight.*

This shows how drastically ideas of correct weight and body styles have changed in less than a century—too little time for our bodies' genetic programming to be sufficiently modified to attain these new ideals. Only a small group of extreme ectomorphs (translation: natural skinnies) can maintain the new body style without considerable dieting effort.

In Eastern and Central Europe, the pleasingly plump look remained popular well into the 1920s and 1930s. A double chin was actually regarded as a sign of beauty in Vienna and points east. That's because a double chin meant that you were rich enough to afford to gorge yourself into status-laden plumpness. Recall the song "If I Were a Rich Man" from *Fiddler on the Roof,* which reflects early twentieth-century Russian ideals of beauty and body style. If he were a rich man, Tevye the milkman sings, he'd make sure his wife would be able to look like a rich man's wife "with a proper double chin."

Russian concepts of beauty and body style haven't changed appreciably since then. The Western taste for thin women is somewhat mystifying to today's Soviet Russians. The peasant appreciation of big women remains a strong determinant of proper body style. Russian women weighing 250 pounds or so think nothing of parading around seaside resorts in bikinis—and no one makes derogatory comments to these bounteous bathing beauties either.

The preference for plumpness is reflected in the Russian language itself. The Russian word for thin is *khudaya,* which is derived from the superlative form of the Russian word for "bad." When the word *khudaya* is applied to a woman, it can have negative connotations, not a compliment at all. And if a Russian woman doesn't look *polniye* (meaning "full" or "plump"), her husband loses status—obviously, he can't be a good breadwinner if his wife is *khudaya,* instead of *polniye.*

However, plumpness had become passé as a body style in most of the Western world by the 1920s. Instead, the boyish flapper look came in. Bosoms were flattened. Knees (preferably bony) were bared. And hips and buttocks were banished to oblivion. The current body style cycle—in which thinness is worshiped—had begun by then. Today the chic body style echoes the dictum of the Duchess of Windsor: "You can never be too rich or too thin."

Still, there are subtle changes in the desirable, slender body shape from year to year. Weight is supposed to be distributed somewhat differently every year or two, in order to make the body style conform to the current clothing style.

"Ideal body shapes have changed tremendously in the past ten years," notes Michael Southgate of Adele Rudstein Mannequins, a firm that manufactures those commercial icons of female beauty, the department-store dummies. "This year," Southgate says, "the ideal body is taller, with a smaller bust, smaller waist, wider shoulders, and longer legs than before."

It's easy to achieve that kind of instant body change with department-store dummies. But it's a different story to try to effect such a substantial shape change on a *real* body, on a real woman. Yet that is precisely what many women try to do. They try to diet and exercise themselves into a new body shape to conform to the current body and clothing styles.

The trouble is that people—men and women alike—often do not take into account their basic, built-in body shapes. They don't consider the built-in genetic, metabolic, and structural factors that make them look like themselves, which is to say unique. Even after arduous dieting, some women attain the "proper" weight for their height and frame, and they'll still have heavy thighs. Some men will diet until they're ready to drop, but they'll still have a bit of a front-porch stomach. These are simply the ways in which these people's bodies are innately programmed to distribute fat and muscle tissues.

One obvious conclusion, then, is that body styles may change, but bodies do not. At least, bodies cannot change drastically, only moderately. If you're not meant to be an extreme endomorph or an extreme mesomorph, all the dieting and exercising in the world will not transform you into that ideal type.

Yet many people are unwilling to accept this obvious conclusion. They torture themselves and the people around them with their unrealistic expectations of how they can make themselves over to look "perfect." But, as we've seen in looking at body styles through history and in various non-Western cultures, there is no single "right" way to look. There is no single "right" weight to be for your height.

As we've noted, beauty or handsomeness is not just in the eye of the beholder. It is in the style of the era, of the culture, of the environmental setting. Today we believe in slenderness, because we have been told it is healthful. And besides, all the popular television and film stars are thin— sometimes to the point of emaciation. They have set the standard for long, lean, and bony as the ideal body style. But if you're short and inclined to be stocky, those body styles are virtually unattainable, even through dint of strenuous exercise and dieting willpower. It is not realistic to expect to be able to remake your body into the current ideal body style.

What then is the *realistic* goal for you? The realistic body-style goal should be becoming the best possible version of you. The best possible *you*, not the best possible imitation of Farrah Fawcett or Robert Redford.

If your body feels healthy, if it functions smoothly, if it feels alive and gives you pleasure, then *that* is an ideal body for you. And it doesn't matter if your waist is "too short" or your hips are "too broad" or your thighs are "too pudgy." What's pudgy or beautiful is merely a matter of different body styles, not of absolutes.

You may be slightly tubby by today's standards, or you may be the "proper" weight and still have the flesh distributed in the "wrong" places. But those are imperfections only because you've picked the wrong era to be overweight in. If you lived in a different era or in a different place, you might be the local equivalent of Venus de Milo or Michelangelo's David.

"We have found fat attractive before; we will do so again. It's our nature," says art historian Anne Hollander, who compiled a massive treatise on the body and clothing, *Seeing Through Clothes.* "Furthermore, health will be on the side of the plump body then, as it is now on the side of the thin. We love to find good reasons for doing things we find aesthetic, and this is no exception."

Think about it again: you're not really fat or ugly or bulgy. You just picked the wrong era to be overweight in. The woman who berates herself for filling out a size 16 can console herself: Rubens, Titian, and Renoir might have considered her delightful-looking, the perfect shape and weight.

By saying it's OK to be overweight (to have a different body style), don't think this gives you permission to go out and eat your way through a half gallon of ice cream single-handed. Being heavy, plump, chubby, *zaftig*—whatever you want to call it—does not mean that gross obesity is OK. Don't abuse your body that way. The realistic body may not be superslender, if that's not your body's innate build. But accepting your own realistic body shape and style does mean that you should try to maximize your health and well-being, that you should take care of yourself by eating nutritiously and moderately and exercising regularly.

The realistic body means that you should take the raw material you've got to work with—your body and its built-in package of genetic, metabolic, environmental, and psychological components—and make that raw material into the best possible finished product. It's a waste of time trying to look like a *Vogue* model when you've never managed to diet below a size 14. It's futile to try to look like a fit and firm tennis star if you are hopelessly unathletic and never looked fit and trim even when you were in high school. But you can make the best out of the body, mind, and spirit you've got to work with.

This brings to mind an old Yiddish folk tale about a man named Yosef who wanted to get to heaven. He did not know how to be virtuous, so he copied every move, every attitude, every opinion of his ideal, Reb Shlomo. When Yosef got to heaven, he told the angels that he was sure he belonged in the celestial city, because "I have made myself over until I'm exactly like Reb Shlomo. I bought the same clothes he did. I ate the same foods he did. I read the same holy books he did. I even prayed in the very same posture as Reb Shlomo."

And so the man thought he would surely enter the Kingdom of Heaven. But then Yosef heard the voice of God say sadly, "You cannot be Reb Shlomo. Only Reb Shlomo can be Reb Shlomo. Instead of trying to be like Reb Shlomo, my son, you should have strived harder to be the best possible you. That is all that God or man can expect of you."

In just the same way, you should have that best-possible-you attitude toward your body and toward the way it looks. Instead of comparing yourself with movie stars, sports heroes, or other celebrities, compare yourself with you. Do you look as good, feel as good about your body today as you did last year or the year before that? If you don't feel comfortable inside your body, no matter what shape that body takes, you won't be happy, nor will you look fantastic.

Your body has unique capacities and capabilities—and unique demands and requirements. Just because you want to look like the currently fashionable body style doesn't mean your body *should* look like that. Maybe your body would function and feel better a bit heavier than the current body style. Maybe your body needs to be thinner than the current body style to function and feel better. If your thighs or your waist are too thick for your tastes, by all means, work on them with shaping exercises.

But don't dislike your body. To dislike your body is to

dislike yourself. The best and only thing you can do in relationship to your body is to be the best possible you.

Your body may not be perfect by today's body-style criteria. But that body is all you've got. Cherish it. Take care of it. Respect it. And most of all, listen to your body. Listen to your body when it tells you at what weight it feels good, at what weight it feels best. Listen to your body when it tells you what kinds of food it needs to work most efficiently and effectively. Listen to your body when it tells you what kinds of physical activities, from jogging to tennis to sex, give it pleasure and make it joyful.

Notice the "faults" of your body's shape and functions. But forgive your body its flaws, its aesthetic imperfections. To reject your body is to reject yourself. And to reject yourself is self-destructive.

Accept and cherish your body. Don't just treat your body as a friend. It's not a friend—your body is *you*.

And ultimately, baby, you're all that you've got.

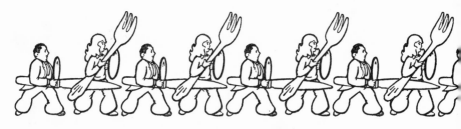

# 16 You Aren't Just What You Eat: Learning Self-Acceptance and Self-Respect

If you are a typical compulsive/emotional eater, you have probably spent a lot of your time being dissatisfied with your weight, with your body, and with your eating habits. You've spent so much time being self-critical that these feelings of self-contempt and loathing have spilled over into all areas of your life and thought. Self-hate has permeated your whole concept of yourself and, thus, infected all your feelings about yourself. Self-hate or self-loathing may become your dominant day-to-day attitude.

To succeed at losing weight, you must first weaken your reasons for eating compulsively and emotionally. But in order to weaken your compulsive eating, you must achieve self-acceptance and self-respect. How do you do this? The first step is linked to your own much-maligned body.

## COME TO TERMS WITH YOUR OWN BODY

If you're going to attain self-acceptance and self-respect, you must learn to separate your feelings about your weight, your body shape, and your eating from your feelings about yourself, your self-image. You are a person with many different abilities, traits, dimensions, and good points—quite apart from your weight or your (over)eating patterns.

Sit down and think about the *good* aspects of your physical appearance. Don't concentrate on your flaws. Zero in on your good points. Your compendium might include items like these: "My hair is shiny and thick," "I have a good complexion," or "I have an attractive face."

Of course, there may still be parts of your body that you think are unsightly or too fat. From now on, don't concentrate on how bad those parts of your body look. Instead, concentrate on how good other parts of your body are. Maybe you have flabby thighs, but you may have a firm stomach. Or you may have pudgy upper arms, but your waist is quite trim.

Take the advice of the popular expression, "I'm not perfect, but parts of me are excellent."

And remember, not even skinny people think their bodies are good-looking in all respects. A thin man may think his arms are too scrawny, his chest too bony. And a thin woman may feel she's too flat-chested or too knobby-kneed. It all goes to show that nobody—no matter how heavy or how thin—thinks he has a perfect body.

Now you're ready to consider your physical *function* good points. We're discussing how your body works here, not how it looks. Consider how well your body serves you every day—how your body takes you where you want to go, how your body functions smoothly and without undue aches or pains. Just for now, forget that you think your legs are too chubby. Right now, be grateful for the fact that those chubby legs can walk for blocks and blocks; be grateful for the fact that you aren't disabled or confined to a wheelchair.

List as many physical-function good points as you can. Some examples: "My body is healthy and strong." "My legs get me where I want to go." "My arms are muscular and can lift heavy loads." "My stomach digests food efficiently and painlessly."

Most people with weight problems dislike their bodies. But what most of us forget is that *we are our bodies*. And if we dislike—or don't accept—our bodies, we can never like or accept ourselves.

American fashion designer Harriet Selwyn remarked, "I once upset a woman customer who told me she couldn't wear anything sleeveless, because she didn't like her arms. I told her, they were *her* arms, and she should like herself."

Selwyn knows what she's talking about when she advises clients to accept their bodies as they are. She herself underwent a mastectomy and had to come to terms with her radically altered body. Instead of hiding in the house, feeling maimed by surgical amputation of a part of her body, Selwyn came to accept her body and herself. She then went on to win fashion awards and greatly expand her business as a designer.

Thus, the first step in achieving a better overall self-image, self-esteem, and self-respect consists of coming to terms with your own body. You must accept your body *as is*. You must learn to be more fully at home living within your own body, accepting it as a unique example of God's handiwork. And recalling your list of physical-function good points, you should also try to view your body as an important personal resource, not as a tiresome, awkward, or unsightly nuisance.

How can you come to terms with your body, when all your life you've felt it was the "wrong" shape?

1. Give up perfectionism when it comes to your body. Don't set unrealistic expectations for what your body can or should look like.

Take heart and realize that even skinnies aren't satisfied with how their bodies are shaped. The exercise director at an elite Los Angeles health spa, which caters to svelte actors, actresses, and models, claims, "No matter how thin or gorgeous they look, they're not happy with their bodies. I've never met *any*body here who thinks his body is perfect just as is."

•  •  •

2. Realize that every body, including yours, is *a work of art*. Somewhere, somewhen in the history of art, some artists considered your body type beautiful. Don't limit your ideas of physical attractiveness to the current era's penchant for super-slimness. Most pre-twentieth-century periods of art glorified much fleshier bodies. When we see these rounder human figures in a work of art by Michelangelo, Giotto, or Brueghel, we find them beautiful. So when you look at your own body—a bit plump by today's limited standards—why don't you apply the same criteria of appreciation to it that you would apply to a similar-looking painting or statue?

Maybe you don't look like a modernistic Giacometti sculpture (a highly elongated, skeletally thin figure). But you may resemble a ripe or monumental figure by Rubens, da Vinci, Monet, Renoir, or Picasso. These artists might have rejoiced in finding a model who was shaped just like you. They might have immortalized your body by turning you into a work of art. So if you could have been a Holbein, Goya, or Rembrandt work of art, how bad-looking can your body actually be? The answer: not bad-looking at all.

If you can, buy a print of an art work that depicts a body type similar to yours. Hang the print on a wall, so that you can look at it every day. That way, you can become accustomed to looking at that kind of body—your kind of body—and considering it admirable and aesthetically pleasing.

3. Stop using derogatory words and terms about your size and shape.

Words make the man, just as surely as clothes do. So if you keep on thinking of yourself and your body in negative, cruel terms, you'll wind up thinking pretty poorly of both your body and yourself.

Find new ways to describe yourself that don't make you feel inferior or inadequate. If you wince at being called "chubby" or "tubby" or "stout," find words or phrases that don't hurt your feelings. For example:

## Bad Descriptions

| | | | |
|---|---|---|---|
| fatso | cow | gross | horse |
| pig | klutz | plump | pudgy |
| ugly | tubby | lardball | hefty |

## Better Descriptions

| | | |
|---|---|---|
| voluptuous | a monumental frame | a person of size |
| solidly built | a Herculean build | generously endowed |
| full-figured | a person of substance | large |

Never underestimate the power of language on your thinking. If you use unflattering or unkind terms for yourself, you will end up thinking badly of yourself. Don't be afraid of using euphemisms. Start right now to make yourself feel better about yourself. A person who feels good about himself gets treated better by other people, too.

## EMPHASIZE ASSETS, NOT ADIPOSE

Now we'll concentrate on building up the inner you, not just the outer, physical you. You can begin this phase of your self-acceptance/self-respect program by starting to compile a **personal assets inventory.**

Take a piece of paper and literally list your good points. Make a list of your abilities, personal assets, and emotional strengths—things that have absolutely nothing to do with your body or physical condition.

The object of this is to convince you that you have a lot more going for you as a human being than your slacks size or whether or not you have a broad bottom.

Here's a sample personal assets inventory that was made by Cathy, a thirty-one-year-old graphic designer:

| | |
|---|---|
| hard worker | intelligent |
| good leader | prompt |
| efficient | artistic |
| trustworthy | sense of humor |
| musical | reliable |
| responsible | capable of earning a good income |

Looking over this personal assets inventory, you can see that Cathy has a lot going for her. She seems to be a pretty special person. And since she's such a special person, Cathy shouldn't dislike herself or feel inferior or want to hide just because she's over her ideal weight.

When you devise your own personal assets inventory, remember to include those personal traits and abilities that you might overlook or take for granted. Don't forget to list things like these:

> kind and caring parent
> good and loyal friend
> devoted son or daughter
> super-homemaker
> considerate, affectionate spouse
> highly sensual, generous lover

In your personal assets inventory, recall all the many things that you do *right*. When you set them all down on a page, you'll discover that the things you do right far outweigh the few things you find wrong with yourself—like your size and shape.

## LOOK BEYOND SUPERFICIAL APPEARANCES

Our society is far too much concerned with what a person looks like, instead of what a person is as a human being. Far too often, we let outward appearances of ourselves and others overshadow many admirable inner qualities that aren't so readily apparent.

Sadly, we tend to judge ourselves and others largely by appearances, by first impressions. And that results in people regarding themselves as 260-pound Glenn did: "When I felt fat, I felt horrible about myself. I hid from social contacts, because I thought people would despise me for my overweight. I felt ugly, so I had no friends, no confidence in myself. I felt I was the scum of the earth." Even though Glenn was a nice person, superficial impressions based on outward appearance poisoned his social contacts and later poisoned his own self-esteem.

If you are ever to live happily with yourself, you must learn to look past the superficial and look within people—including yourself. Friends and relatives of compulsive/emotional eaters would help immeasurably if they, too, could learn to look past superficial appearances and more fully appreciate the human being within the body.

Perhaps we should update the old saying "Pretty is as pretty does." Modernized, that might translate to: "Thin is as thin does. Fat is as fat does." This doesn't mean that we're advising people to get fat or to completely let go and overeat constantly, using compulsive/emotional eating as an excuse. By all means, keep on trying to get down to your desired weight and stay there.

But also realize that thin people are not automatically superior to you. Thin people are not better than you are; they are just different. You shouldn't hold people in high regard and envy them just because they are slim. You, a person with a weight problem, may have vastly superior talents, intelligence, abilities, and emotional depth. This can easily be discerned if people will just look past superficial appearances and stop judging a person's worth largely by outward appearance.

## VALUE YOURSELF

To avoid self-destructive or self-loathing behavior and depression, you must learn to value yourself. Most people don't feel they have any worth as people until others value them. Feelings of worth and value must come from within ourselves. Worth and value cannot be bestowed on us by others' regard. Nor can our personal worth and value be taken away from us simply because others don't appreciate us.

What this means, in essence, comes down to that current cliché: Be your own best friend. Or at least, be your own close buddy.

One important part of valuing yourself is to emphasize your successes and deemphasize or forget your shortcomings and failures. Get into the habit of regarding yourself as a winner, not a loser.

Think like a winner, too. Just because you have a weight problem, you shouldn't feel as if you're personally bankrupt as a human being. Your weight shouldn't make or break you as a person, least of all in your own estimation of yourself.

One person who has obviously learned to value herself is Elizabeth Taylor, who has been widely admired as one of the great beauties of our era. Yet in recent years, Taylor has quite noticeably put on weight. Part of her growing weight problem may be the onset of middle age. But perhaps Taylor has also come to terms with herself and achieved a kind of self-acceptance and self-esteem that exists independently of her weight.

As Taylor's current husband, United States Senator John Warner, told an interviewer, Elizabeth Taylor now has "an attitude of 'I am what I am, and I have a few pounds. So be it.' " Warner went on to say, "I think the important aspects of Elizabeth Taylor are her intellect, her humor, her warmth, as opposed to her physical beauty. A few pounds haven't detracted as far as I am concerned."

## PICK FRIENDS, NOT ENEMIES

Don't spend a lot of time with people who put you down or criticize you solely because of your weight. These people aren't friends; they are enemies. When they tear you down, they assault your already fragile sense of self-acceptance and self-respect.

Show your self-respect by standing up to these people. Tell them that there's more to a person than just physical looks. (You'll believe this yourself, too, if you've done your homework earlier in this chapter by compiling a personal assets inventory.)

Put these critical people who downgrade you into their places by telling them they're weightist bigots. (Consult the next chapter, "Weightism: Prejudice in a Thin-Obsessed

Society," so you'll understand bigotry based on weight more clearly.)

If these "friends" don't take your hints, suggestions, and declarations that they're being destructive in their critical comments toward you, then drop them. Friends like that you can do without. When you like yourself better, you won't need to hold on to unkind friends who make you feel inferior and inadequate.

## OUT WITH GUILT AND SHAME

Guilt and shame about your weight problem are counter-productive. Don't let yourself indulge in guilt or shame about your shape or size or how much you "should" weigh. Guilt and shame won't prod you into losing weight. On the contrary, these self-flagellating emotions will just make you feel so bad about yourself that you'll end up self-destructively overeating.

## DAYDREAM POSITIVELY

Try to practice positive, controlled daydreaming. This should help you to feel good, to feel positive, about yourself.

The technique of positive, controlled daydreaming has been used with considerable success as part of weight-loss programs supervised by Dr. Frances Stern, a clinical psychologist, who is chief of the Institute for Behavioral Awareness in Springfield, New Jersey. Dr. Stern's technique is similar to controlled daydreaming systems taught in hypnosis, Silva Mind Control, and autosuggestion.

To daydream in the controlled, positive manner, first get into a comfortable, relaxed position, preferably in a quiet room by yourself. Close your eyes. Then proceed to relive a positive, "up" experience of your own. This should be an incident that made you feel really good about yourself. The suitable positive daydreaming experience to recall might be the day you got a promotion or won an award, the time your friends threw you a surprise birthday party, the day you graduated or got married.

Whatever specific episode you select for your positive daydream, you must try to recall every detail, even the tiniest. Recall what the temperature was, how the air smelled, what you wore, how you smiled or laughed.

The concept behind the positive, controlled daydream is to remember, vividly and in detail, something that made you feel proud and happy to be you. The daydream will reinforce and expand your growing feelings of self-esteem and self-respect by letting you dwell on positive things you have done. Try to make this pride and feeling of accomplishment and self-worth spread to all areas of your consciousness.

For maximum effectiveness, repeat your positive, controlled daydream once or twice a day for at least two weeks. Let those good feelings about yourself be repeated until they really sink in!

## BE KIND TO YOURSELF

Show yourself as much compassion and kindness as you show other people.

Self-compassion is largely absent in people who are compulsive/emotional eaters—they despise themselves too much. Usually, compulsive/emotional eaters are much kinder and generally nicer to other (thinner) people than they are to themselves.

Don't just shower your family, friends, and co-workers with compassion and affection. Shower a little of that compassion and affection on yourself for a change. Don't hold back—you *deserve* it.

Behaving with kindness and compassion toward yourself isn't selfishness. Rather, it is sensible—a matter of self-preservation and self-enhancement.

## DIET FOR SOMEONE YOU LOVE

Feeling better about yourself as a person may very likely make your next stab at dieting go more easily. You may actually be more successful at losing weight and keeping it off once you've achieved a fair degree of self-acceptance and self-respect.

Why should this be so?

Because this time you'll be trying to help a person you really love, admire, and respect—yourself.

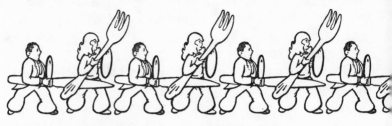

# 17  Weightism: Prejudice
## in a Thin-Obsessed Society

What is weightism?

Everyone knows what racism is, what sexism is. These are ignorant, irrational prejudices held against members of minority, or even majority, groups. But did you ever consider that overweight Americans are a minority group, too? The overweight constitute over 40 percent of the nation's population. And the ignorant, irrational prejudices held against the overweight are nothing more than bigotry against an oppressed minority group.

Society has grown more accepting of other oppressed minority groups. Legislation has been passed to aid them. They benefit from special programs in both the private and public sectors of the economy. At the very least, consciousness of racism, sexism, ageism, and other prejudices has increased among the general public. But hardly anybody is aware of weightism.

Weightism is prejudice against the overweight just because they *are* overweight. Weightism is so ingrained in this pro-thin society that we aren't even aware that weightism *is* a prejudice. Weightism is one of the few prejudices that no one is embarrassed to practice.

Believe it or not, you practice weightism every day—

even if you yourself are overweight. We have accepted that black can be beautiful. But how many of us have accepted that heavy can be handsome (or beautiful), too?

We have been educated over the years to abhor racism. The media have exhorted that blacks, Hispanics, and other people of color can do the job, can work as efficiently and effectively as the white majority. Even when people do act prejudiced against other minorities, they *know* that they're behaving in a bigoted manner. Maybe they even feel ashamed of themselves or embarrassed for behaving in a socially unacceptable way. But hardly anyone ever gives a second thought to how utterly wrong and bigoted they are when they practice weightism.

The overweight in this society are victims of arbitrary standards and commercial conditioning, of an entire social and media structure that trumpets the glories of thinness. The society's underlying prejudice against overweight is expressed in countless ways (many of them are enumerated later in this chapter). But a telling attitude reveals this society's implicit weightism: underweight is considered a medical problem, while overweight is considered a sign of emotional weakness.

The overweight person is victimized in this society. He or she is often denied employment and job advancement because of overweight, is denied any vestige of dignity or pride in his or her body, is denied many social and sexual opportunities. The overweight are criticized, scorned, and reviled because of their weight alone. They are stigmatized from the first disapproving glance of a stranger.

The members of this oppressed minority group, the overweight, usually lead lives of mild to severe anguish and self-loathing because of the continual expressions of weightist prejudice to which they are subjected.

The overweight are victims, often denied the opportunities for advancement and happiness which most Americans take for granted. These oppressed people come in all colors, from all ethnic and religious groups, all levels of education and economic class. The only thing they truly have in common is their overweight—and their victimization by weightist prejudice.

## OVERWEIGHT PEOPLE AS SOCIAL LEPERS

In some ways, today's overweight people are the twentieth century's equivalent of the ancient world's shunned and abused lepers.

Both obesity and leprosy are highly *visible* disorders. Unlike alcoholism, compulsive gambling, or drug addiction, the dread affliction of overweight is easily *seen*.

Like lepers, the overweight are shunned socially. Weightist prejudices make it seem as if overweight might be contagious. Or, more likely, weightist bigots feel that hanging around with overweight people—people who have low social status as overweights, despite their economic class and/or achievements—might bring down their status, too. Associating with the overweight confers lower social status on their thin friends and lovers. If you don't believe this, consider how most Americans would snicker at a thin man seen dating a woman fifty pounds overweight.

In ancient times, the leper was regarded with horror as "unclean, unclean." Today the heavier person is similarly regarded with a mixture of horror and derision as "fat, fat."

Of course, the very words *fat, plump, chubby, hefty, large,* and *stout* have become synonyms for (at best) unattractive and (at worst) ugly. Nobody envies the fat man, but many people try to exploit him.

## WEIGHTISM IN ACTION

"Hey, fatso!"
"She looks like a house."
"What a gut he's got, hanging down in front!"
"Honey, you've gained so much weight, you look just like a baby elephant."

260

"Her backside is so big, it looks like a train followed by a caboose."

"What a beer belly! You look like you're pregnant, fella."

These are the kinds of weightist remarks that overweight people are subjected to. These are prejudices, ridicule aimed at people because they're minority group members. You wouldn't tell somebody that he's "too black" or he's "got a great sense of rhythm, just like all your people." These are obviously prejudiced, racist remarks. Yet most people would not believe they're weightist bigots when they inform someone that he's "too fat" or "jolly, just like all heavy people."

Supposedly, inside every fat man, there's a thin man trying to get out. But when you consider the amount of weightist prejudice directed against the overweight person in this society, you could amend that aphorism to "Inside every fat man, there's a human being begging to be left in peace."

It is taken for granted that overweight people will be ridiculed in this society. The nonthin person must constantly battle against the weightist prejudice inherent in our thin-indoctrinated society. Eventually, most overweight people do succumb to weight problems—but the weight problem isn't really how many pounds they're over the "ideal weight." The real weight problem is the stigma and ridicule loaded on them by the bigoted members of a society that harbors and even nurtures deep, illogical prejudices against the overweight.

In the chapter "Culture 'Talks' Thin," we saw how this culture extols the virtues of slenderness and propagandizes for thin and against fat. And we've seen in other chapters how our attitudes about the "right" body shape and weight are *not* absolutes but are really culturally determined by the currently fashionable body styles.

Even when you understand these factors, it isn't much consolation for the person who is overweight in this society. That's because in most people's minds, there's an unconscious, weightist equation that springs into action when they're evaluating an overweight person. And that equation is:

$$\text{Overweight} = \text{an undisciplined, ugly person}$$
$$= \text{an unworthy person}$$

On the other hand, thinness is associated with desirability, competence, beauty, even goodness. Being thin gives an individual a built-in edge over the overweight. Thin people are automatically considered OK, considered worthwhile human beings, no matter how rotten, superficial, or commonplace they actually may be. But the overweight person must constantly *prove* his worth in this society where self-worth is linked with outward physical appearance—not with thoughts, feelings, or actions.

The rampant weightist prejudice always present in this society has led to self-hate for many heavy or even average-weight people. They feel they're somehow inferior, because they can't keep their weight down to acceptably thin levels. They are filled with self-hatred, which is really society's prejudice against them turned inward.

## WEIGHTIST MYTHS

Prejudice against the overweight is so widespread in affluent Western society that this bigotry can be found in virtually every aspect of daily life, so deeply ingrained that a whole anti-overweight mythology has developed.

Among the many commonly held myths (and remember, these statements are myths, not facts) are such familiar ideas as:

- Overweight people have no self-control.
- Overweight people are too irresponsible to keep themselves in shape, so how can they manage a business/home/office/club effectively?
- Overweight people are greedy and selfish; that's how they got overweight in the first place.
- Overweight people are stupid.
- Overweight people are slobs.

262

- Overweight people smell bad, because they sweat so much more than other people.
- Overweight people don't look "right" as executives or doctors or lawyers or ministers.
- Overweight people are so fat and jolly and full of laughs that they're not sensitive when you kid them about their weight.
- Overweight people aren't interested in sex, and they couldn't perform right, even if they were interested. You know, they just got fat to hide from sex and sexual advances.

All these outlandish statements are blithely accepted by many people in this culture, because they've become such common, ingrained stereotypes about the overweight.

**None of these stereotypes is true.**

If you said the same things about other minority groups, such as blacks, Hispanics, or women, you'd be accused of prejudice. If you utter these myths about the overweight, however, you're not considered prejudiced at all. You're merely considered to be displaying folk wisdom. But if you believe such stereotypes, you're a weightist bigot.

And if you yourself are an overweight person, you've probably swallowed all these anti-fat prejudices, too, and have been mercilessly criticizing yourself for looking that way. Which leads to self-hate, which leads to depression or anxiety attacks, which leads to overeating, which leads to more overweight. It's a vicious cycle, in which the oppressed (the overweight) become their own worst oppressors.

## THE ROOTS OF WEIGHTIST PREJUDICE

To break this pattern of self-hate, stemming from internalizing society's prejudices against the overweight, it's important to understand the roots of weightism. You have to raise your consciousness about the severe discrimination overweight people are subjected to. In this way, you'll better understand your own superficial and often callous treatment of yourself and other overweight persons. And, you can start to understand precisely how the overweight came to be regarded as second-class citizens.

Prejudice against the overweight begins in childhood. The overweight child is often subjected to jibes and taunts about his weight.

> "Fatty, fat, two by four
> Can't fit through the classroom door."

That's a traditional schoolyard chant. Any overweight child who is subjected to ridicule like this from his schoolmates will naturally begin to think there's something wrong with him as a person.

The overweight child soon learns that being heavy is terrible, ugly, and embarrassing. Children sling around unkind labels like "fatty," "chubs," "gross," "horse," and "pig" at the heavier child, who often becomes a scapegoat because of his size.

"I got called fatty so much in grade school that I got this self-image of myself as enormously fat," says one now-svelte young woman. "I was stunned when I looked over some old snapshots of myself as a little kid. I wasn't so fat. I was just slightly chubby and, in fact, a pretty damn cute kid at that. And all those years, I thought I was enormous and grotesque because of what the other kids said."

Why do other children pick on the overweight child? Partly because children will react to anyone who is somewhat different from the norm. But mostly because children learn their parents' values, their parents' prejudices. Just as children learn racism and sexism at home, they learn weightism at home, too.

The overweight child can have his self-image and self-esteem badly (and possibly permanently) damaged by casually cruel childhood name-calling.

What children and all too many adults don't realize is that names like "fatty" and "piggy" are just as vile and just as prejudiced when used against the overweight as are terms like "nigger," "wop," and "spic" when directed against other minority groups. None of these terms is acceptable. By now, most people are enlightened enough to censor themselves against saying such offensive words. But how many people in this thin-obsessed society are aware enough to censor themselves before making cruel remarks about the overweight?

Not the well-known actress who declared on a network television talk show that "fat people pollute the environment. There should be fat-catchers to haul them away, so the rest of us don't have to look at them." Her remark was greeted with chuckles from the studio audience, not with gasps of indignation at such blatant prejudice being expressed so openly.

Although weightism's first effects are felt in childhood, the prejudice inflicts more damaging punishments as the heavier individual grows older. College admissions practices, for instance, are often discriminatory toward overweight applicants.

Studies showed that a heavy high-school graduate faces substantial discrimination when applying for college admission. According to a Harvard School of Public Health research project, this weightism becomes most severe when the overweight student is a female and has to come for a personal interview—and is seen in full girth—before an admissions decision is made.

Weightist bias by college admissions officers cuts the chances of the noticeably overweight applicant's acceptance in half! These findings were reported by Dr. Natalie Allon, a Hofstra University sociologist.

At least one university has openly discriminated against overweight students even after they have been admitted. Oral Roberts University in Tulsa, Oklahoma, demanded that every student with "10 percent excess fat" had to go into a weight-reduction program. Those who did not participate in such a reducing program faced suspension from college (regardless of their academic standing), as did those who did not lose the required pound per week on the diet. Four students were suspended for overweight—a reason that had nothing to do with their scholastic records.

In another case, a fourth-year woman medical student

at a large midwestern state university was expelled for reasons that included her being overweight. As this woman told the *New York Times*, ". . . some students tried to make my weight an issue [in my expulsion]. I'm heavy, but I'm in the right shape—with a few extra inches. . . . Some students and faculty said they didn't feel I look like a doctor [should]."

## WEIGHTISM AT WORK

The prejudice against the overweight is expressed in many overt and subtle ways in the working world. The overweight job seeker is at a disadvantage; most employers prefer to hire thin or "normal-weight" people. This judgment is based on the false stereotype that the overweight lack self-control, willpower, ambition, drive, and organization.

"Weight is also considered for jobs [as] typists, file clerks, receptionists, and secretaries, where the public might form an impression of the company by the employees on display," Dr. Natalie Allon said, explaining her research findings. "But these considerations are only admitted off the record."

A large employment agency's survey found that over the years, the agency had received thousands of requests from employers for "thin" people to fill job vacancies. But the employment agency found it had received only one request in twenty-five years for a "plump" person to fill a job. And that job was with a firm that manufactured large-size men's clothes.

Many state, county, and municipal governments in the United States have hiring guidelines which preclude hiring people who are more than a certain percentage above the "desirable" weights for their heights. Health reasons and lack of adequate insurance coverage for overweight workers are frequently given as justifications for this kind of overt discrimination. Often the real reason for rejecting overweight job applicants is sheer weightism: overweight people aren't deemed "attractive enough" to work in the office.

Insurance coverage is one of the most frequently cited

reasons for companies' flatly rejecting qualified job applicants who are overweight. Many corporations' medical insurance plans for employees exclude overweight individuals. The corporations solve this problem of uninsured workers: they just don't hire any people who are overweight and who wouldn't automatically be given group coverage rates by the insurance companies. Simple solution—weightist solution.

Once hired, overweight people are typically not advanced as quickly or as far up the corporate ladder as are thinner people, another personnel-agency study revealed. The overweight are seldom found in top-echelon positions in corporate America. Very few chief executive officers of large, publicly held corporations are much more than ten pounds overweight. The problem isn't that overweight people can't handle top executive positions. The problem is that overweight people usually aren't considered for such positions. Maybe big corporations' boards of directors have the same weightist mentality as most personnel departments. They all "think thin" and punish the pudgy through their discriminatory hiring and promotional patterns.

## WEIGHTISM AND POLITICS

Because of weightism, fat people in the United States carry less and less weight in politics. Few noticeably overweight candidates are nominated, even fewer get elected. That's because the conventional wisdom among professional political analysts is that an overweight candidate will receive fewer votes than a thin candidate, irrespective of their stands on the issues.

That's why most politicians' campaign managers strongly urge their candidates to lose weight. When the candidate becomes thinner, the voters supposedly perceive the same politician as more vigorous, more youthful, more capable, and more energetic. Another case of less is more: less weight equals more votes.

One Washington columnist, Daniel S. Greenberg, has

gone so far as to say, "No fat man can be elected president of the United States." Voter prejudice against overweight people is so pervasive, Greenberg believes, that a fat or substantially overweight candidate would be defeated at the polls by the scales.

## WEIGHTISM IMPAIRS SOCIAL AND SEX LIVES

Of course, many overweight individuals triumph over prejudice and wind up holding good jobs and earning excellent incomes. They succeed—despite discrimination. But the social scene is cruelly prejudiced against the overweight.

The overweight teenage girl is far less likely to be asked out on a date than her thinner counterpart. Because she's overweight, a girl is considered a less desirable date. Her appearance brands her boyfriends with guilt by association —if they're so hard up that they date a fatso, then they must be turkeys themselves.

Similarly, the overweight teenage boy becomes shy about asking girls out, because his weight sets him up for a more-than-usual share of rejections. Of course, if he's a heavyset star football player or wrestler, then bulk becomes a status symbol and may help in getting dates.

But by and large, in the adolescent social world, overweight confers very low status on the overweight and on those who date them.

This anti-heavies attitude carries over into adult social life. At dating bars, for instance, the primary concern in picking up a partner for some small talk and some possible sex play is: do they look good? "Looking good" is, of course, defined as thinness. Heavier people have fewer opportunities to socialize and get into love relationships than do thinner people of comparable emotional and financial desirability.

Overweights are used to being considered "dogs" or wallflowers. It's their social role in a culture that's virulently prejudiced against overweight individuals. Indeed, studies have demonstrated that people tend to dislike or to be condescending toward the overweight—just on the basis of their appearance. And these thin people discriminate socially against the overweight and are not ashamed of their weightist discrimination. No wonder overweight people feel like social outcasts. They are.

Of course, there are *some* men and women who prefer their sex partners fat and fleshy. These fatophiles are unflatteringly termed "chubby chasers," and they themselves are often subjected to ridicule and ribbing by their friends. "One of my friends has a thing about going out with blue-eyed blondes," a self-confessed chubby chaser recounted. "He thinks that's perfectly normal; that's his preference. My preference is going out with big women, very heavy women, and my friend thinks I'm nuts. Most people think I'm nuts. But I figure, how is liking big women so different from liking blue-eyed blondes?"

Heavy bodies in this culture are not considered suitable for making love. Sexual intercourse, for many people, has come to mean a kind of athletic demonstration, which should be engaged in only by the slim and supple. The nudity involved in sexual activities is another drawback for many overweight people who have directed weightist prejudices against themselves. These people are often too ashamed of their fleshy bodies to show themselves freely to their sex partners, much less to engage in relaxed and uninhibited sexual play.

Some overweight people do, in fact, want to avoid sex and use their fatness as a shield. The Fortress of Fat eating personality type is just such a person (see Chapter 8). But Fortresses of Fat are *not* the rule among the overweight.

## DEMOLISHING MYTHS ABOUT OVERWEIGHT AND SEX

Heavier people may get fewer opportunities for varied sex partners than their thinner counterparts because of the prevailing social prejudice against the overweight. But most overweight people enjoy and crave sex just as much as thin people do. And unless the degree of overweight is very considerable indeed, overweight should cause no impairment of sexual functioning or potential pleasures.

Some overweight men think they have unusually small genitals; they dread intercourse because of shame. They don't want to reveal to their partner(s) that they're "underendowed." But for the most part, these men don't have abnormally small sex organs at all. Rather, their genitals may be partially hidden by flesh. Or their genitals may only *seem* small when contrasted with their large overall body size.

And far from being afraid of sex or being sexually frigid, overweight women are shown by several studies to be more highly sexed than women of average or thin body builds.

"Nobody loves a fat girl, but, oh, how a fat girl can love," went the old vaudeville song. In his book *Sex and the Overweight Woman*, Dr. Eugene Scheimann claimed that the overweight woman is a better sex partner than her thinner sister. Scheimann stated that plump or heavy women might have more "insatiable" appetites for both food and sex. To extend the analogy, Scheimann thought that overweight women might relish experimentation in both these areas of sensuality—eating and making love.

Another study, conducted at Chicago's Michael Reese Hospital by Dr. Ronald A. Schwartz and Dr. William G. Shipman, showed that obese married women have sexual relationships with their husbands just as often as nonobese married women. So much for the myth of sexual avoidance or frigidity among heavier women. Even more surprisingly, Schwartz and Shipman found that the overweight women expressed the desire to engage in sex more frequently than they presently did. In contrast, the nonobese wives in this study said they wished they could have sex *less* frequently. The researchers ultimately concluded that the overweight married women were "more highly sexed" than their thinner counterparts.

Many overweight people report that they overeat when they feel underloved or sexually frustrated. So their overweight may, in part, be traced to sexual desire, not to sexual avoidance or frigidity.

Others studies have demonstrated that when women lose substantial amounts of weight, their sex drives often slow down, too; these formerly heavy women find their sexual demands taper off until they reach the lower sexual-demand level of the typical thin women. Here reducing the lard seems to be linked to reducing the lust.

## CLOTHING FOR GOOD MEASURE

Social prejudice against the overweight extends outside the bedroom and into the dressing room. Although over 40 percent of Americans are overweight, really attractive and trendy clothing has been available only in smaller sizes until quite recently. About 25 million women wear sizes over 16, yet the clothing industry made it almost impossible for these women to buy colorful and stylish clothes until the past few years. That's when the thinness-oriented fashion designers finally came to grips with the economic facts of life: while the rest of the apparel industry usually has sales increases below 7 percent annually, companies which market clothes for heavier women were reporting sales increases of 15 to 25 percent annually.

Why the boom in larger-size clothes? Because there are more larger-size women to wear and buy them. The *New York Times* cites statistics that show "more than half of American women wear size 14 and up." *Newsweek* pins it down even more precisely: "One-third of American women now wear upwards of a size 16—an outfit that generally suits a 38–30–38 figure."

The statistics on larger-size clothing for men roughly parallels the statistics for women. If you are heavy, you are no longer alone in America. But you are still discriminated against in purchasing clothes.

Many clothing designers still feel it is impossible to be both fashionable and overweight. One American designer who limits his women's couture line to sizes no bigger than

271

12 explains his small-size rationale this way: "I don't think it's possible for a woman who's a size 14 or 16 to look stylish. The clothes won't lie right on her; too many bulges, too much bulk. My clothes should really only be worn by a slim woman, preferably tallish, with long, graceful legs." Which does tend to exclude a sizable portion of the female population.

These weightist attitudes are drilled into fashion designers from their earliest days in design school. There weightism is a vital though unrecognized part of the curriculum. An outstanding fashion-design student at the Parsons School of Design (one of the most prestigious training grounds for the fashion industry) frankly expressed his education in weightism: "In design school, we're taught to draw and to design for the tall, slender, lovely, elegant woman. I wouldn't feel right designing for a heavier person." The design student actually giggled at this point, noting, "Heavy people look funny to me. I try not to think about the way they look. It's not aesthetically acceptable."

These statements are weightism at its most blatant. Would the Parsons student *dare* to talk in the same prejudiced manner about blacks, Puerto Ricans, or WASPs? Would he say that because they are black, brown, or lily white, their physical appearance was not "aesthetically acceptable"? Elegance and loveliness should not be measured by the pound but by a person's attitude, style, and bearing.

Still, buying clothes is not an easy task for the person who wears larger sizes. "It's hard to shop when there's nothing in the store that'll fit," quips one plump stand-up comedienne. "I have to take two size 11's and sew them together."

Larger-size clothes for men, women, and children are relegated to ghettos in major department stores. The overweight buyer thus suffers from segregation—separate but unequal facilities. Although substantial numbers of men and women wear bigger sizes, they have to ferret out the department stores' "half size" (for women) or "big men's" sections. These large-size departments are often drably decorated and cramped, hidden in out-of-the-way corners of the department stores, as if they were the retailers' equivalent of idiot children hidden in the attic. Many retailers still seem to be trying to pretend that big sizes and big-sized customers don't exist.

Many overweight men and women report incident after incident of being humiliated and ridiculed by clothing sales personnel, because these customers were too large to fit into the smaller, more fashionable sizes.

There are, of course, national chains and local specialty stores that cater to overweight clientele. Once again, this consumer ghettoization results in separate but unequal facilities. Chains like Lane Bryant and Roaman's have prospered by offering large women a wide range of clothing, though until recently the uniform for the heavy woman was the ubiquitous dark-colored double-knit pantsuit.

However, many of the big-size customers complain about the way the new styles are cut and designed. "Most of the manufacturers of half-size and large-size clothes have no idea of what looks well on a bigger woman," one size-18½ woman griped. "The clothes often aren't flattering. They make you look boxy and square, instead of showing that we do have curves and shapes."

Another irony many customers of the large-size-clothing stores notice: most models in the Lane Bryant and Roaman's catalogues are built like conventional models—slim and long—not like the people who will actually wear the larger-sized clothes. A few noticeably plump models are used in advertising larger-size clothes; this is a relatively recent innovation. But these heavyish models are definitely in the minority, in both print ads and live fashion shows. Some large-size manufacturers seem to use plump models for shock value in their print advertising campaigns.

What's the reason for this apparent prejudice against the overweight models, even by the stores and clothing manufacturers who cater to them? It seems to be the prejudice of the overweight consumers themselves against the heavier models. "We tried it and discovered that our customers just didn't want to buy clothes that we photographed on heavy models," remarked a marketing executive at one big-sizes clothing chain. "I guess our customers don't want to face reality—that they'll look heavy no matter what clothes they wear."

In this instance, overweight people are helping to discriminate against themselves. Well, why not? The overweight are a part of this society, too. They've swallowed the cultural conditioning that slim is good and heavy is bad, that any degree of overweight carries a stigma along with the excess poundage.

Patronizing the large-sizes stores in itself carries a certain stigma. "Walking down the street with a Lane Bryant shopping bag is like an announcement to the world that you're too big to fit into regular clothes, that you're no longer a normal human being, that you're a fat freak," lamented one overweight woman, a magazine editor. "It got me so embarrassed that I started calling Lane Bryant 'the house of shame.' If I had to buy clothes there, I'd sneak in through a side entrance, so nobody would see me go in. And I'd bring a Bloomingdale's bag to carry home my purchases. I was just too humiliated to walk through the streets with a Lane Bryant's shopping bag, announcing to the world that I'm big, big, big."

Of course, not every large-size person feels so stigmatized by Lane Bryant. Many are grateful that they have a convenient source of clothing in their sizes. But the person who patronizes specialty stores for larger sizes often faces ridicule besides everyday weightism.

Like the suburban juvenile delinquent who eschewed violent assaults. His assaults were psychological ones, on the obese: "I used to stand in front of the fat lady shop and laugh real loud as all the tubby women went in. It *destroyed* them!" Maybe that's an extreme example. But it is indicative of the disrespect this society regularly levels at its heavier citizens.

## HELPERS OR PERSECUTORS?

Well, you may say, the fashion industry is the bastion of thinness. They're the biggest propagandists for the slenderness cult. But the overweight face prejudice even from their supposed champions.

Very often, diet experts are the worst persecutors of the overweight. These persecutors may be instructors in the group weight-loss programs (i.e., Weight Watchers and its imitators) and weight-loss clubs. These people all too frequently degrade and debase the self-esteem of the overweight individuals they're supposed to help.

These persecutors—often former fatties themselves—pound the idea into heavier people's heads that because they're overweight, they're not as good as thinner people, that the overweight must respect slim people more than they do themselves just because those people are thin. The overweight are dunned into believing that they are emotional and moral weaklings because they weigh too much. This is simply another way in which the overweight are taught to regard themselves as second-class citizens—and as second-class human beings.

Some of the harshest persecutors of the overweight are people in the medical profession. Physicians are by no means exempt from the cultural prejudices against overweight. They often verbally flagellate their heftier patients, trying to make guilt and shame integral parts of their reducing plans, and generally making their patients feel that being overweight is a terrible disgrace.

Some physicians try to bully their patients into losing weight. Others are so contemptuous of the overweight that these doctors give up on their heavy patients. A survey conducted by the Health and Weight Program at the Johns Hopkins Medical Institutions revealed that 25 percent of the physicians surveyed "don't even want to bother" with fat patients.

Doctors often justify their bullying of overweight patients —insisting that they "lose weight or else"—on the grounds that overweight can lead to or aggravate heart disease, diabetes, and other serious conditions. Most doctors automatically assume that losing weight will be beneficial to the patient. But that may not necessarily be true. Dr. Theodore Isaac Rubin, a psychiatrist who has often worked with overweight people, believes that staying thin may, in some ways, actually be physically harmful to people who are genetically programmed to run to fat: "For people on the heavy side to maintain extreme thinness brings in a stress factor that can become quite destructive."

As associate director of the obesity program of the Karen Horney Clinic in New York City, Dr. Douglas H. Ingram works with many overweight individuals. He has pointed out that doctors who cite the medically harmful effects of overweight are supporting a position that is "tenuous" at best. "The scientific medical literature on the subject of obesity reveals too many contradictions, too much uncertainty, too little factual, reproducible data in support of statements that hold non-massive obesity contributory to physical illnesses," Dr. Ingram has written. "Most doctors, true, agree that weight reduction is an important part of the treatment of certain ills. Yet we cannot show that healthy fat people have better chances of remaining healthy if they lose weight and keep it off." Ingram calls for "at least some skepticism" about the medical advantages of weight reduction.

Supporting this viewpoint are findings which show that being moderately overweight will not shorten your life span —if you don't have other health problems. Dr. Reubin Andres, clinical director of the National Institute on Aging at the Gerontology Research Center of Baltimore, comments, "Being 10 or 20 or even 30 percent over your 'desirable' weight does not lead to a shortened life in the middle-aged or elderly. Several studies have failed to show obesity having the effect of shortening life." Dr. Andres admits, "We don't understand this. It's really surprising."

However, most American-trained physicians maintain a

very simplistic attitude: overweight is bad and should be eliminated as quickly as possible. And similarly, they have simplistic views about why the overweight individual has a weight problem: he is believed to be self-indulgent or neurotic or perverse. Very few doctors have adequate training in nutrition, much less training in the causes and cures of obesity. And exceedingly few physicians take a holistic viewpoint regarding the treatment and/or management of obesity.

Most doctors ignore or discount the cultural and psychological factors that are involved in overeating and, consequently, in weight gain. For instance, a physician with a thriving "diet practice" with offices in Manhattan, Queens, and Long Island purports to treat obesity. Yet he ignores the social and psychological aspects of the condition. When interviewed, this doctor is frankly contemptuous of his overweight patients, though he is not contemptuous of taking their money in fees. This "diet doctor" thinks that "overweight people just lack discipline and need to be hounded into willpower."

Another (very expensive) doctor who specializes in weight control says he does his job by handing his patients diet menus for 1,200 calories a day and by giving them "little lectures." The doctor describes his lectures as "inspirational," but a former patient describes them as "sadistic bullying." This physician bluntly states, "It's not my job to comfort them or to deal with their neurotic behavior. I can't help it if they don't have willpower."

Although he deals almost exclusively with the problems of overweight, this man shows no compassion and very little insight into the emotional blocks and cultural conditioning that helped make his patients heavy. This physician is, in fact, a weightist, a prejudiced person, though he doesn't even know it. And this doctor is not atypical.

Many doctors are frankly scornful or critical of their overweight patients. And these weightist attitudes and methods don't help the overweight patients to lose weight.

Instead, having cultural prejudice against heaviness reinforced by physicians may actually make it much more difficult for the overweight person to lose weight. Society's prejudices against the overweight have already made many overweight people feel ostracized. Consequently, they often become shy, lacking in self-esteem, and highly self-critical. The abusive or contemptuous physician may reinforce the patient's already low opinion of himself. And this may trigger yet another wave of self-destructive and/or self-pitying eating binges.

Perhaps the doctors' unconscious prejudice against the overweight is one significant reason why the medical profession has been so abysmally unsuccessful in dealing with obesity, much less curing it. Maybe physicians don't have the answers or the programs to fight obesity successfully because physicians, by and large, are too weightist to deal with overweight people and their problem in a manner that combines scientific objectivity and humane compassion.

Although the United States Senate Select Committee on Nutrition and Human Need reported that overweight is a national epidemic in America and the nation's most widespread health problem, very little federal money has gone into obesity research. CBS News has estimated that more money is spent on fad diets and fad weight-loss regimes "than on all research for a cure to obesity combined." Through the National Institutes of Health, the federal government supports only one full-fledged, multidisciplinary center for obesity research and treatment. This lone program (at St. Luke's Hospital Center in New York City) did not begin operations until 1974.

Consequently, doctors have only fragmentary knowledge with which to treat their overweight patients' conditions. No wonder the medical system fails to get good results. No wonder people diet more and end up weighing more, on average. As one cynical overweight man noted, "You've got a better chance to be cured of cancer than to lose weight and keep it off!"

Maybe the relative lack of obesity research also stems from weightism. Obesity research certainly couldn't be considered a glamorous area of medicine or science. Of course not—weightism tells us that anything connected with overweight is *de facto* unglamorous, even slightly ludicrous.

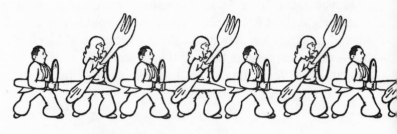

# 18  Fighting Weightism

From all sides, the overweight person in this society finds himself engulfed in weightism, attacked by subtle and not-so-subtle antiweight ridicule and discrimination.

"If somebody were walking down the street, and they were crippled or blind or black, nobody would tell them to change the way they looked," an overweight woman remarks ruefully. "But because I'm heavy, total strangers feel free to walk up to me on the street and tell me in really strong, vicious language that I should be ashamed of myself, that I should lose weight, that I'm creating a public eyesore."

Most people don't get quite so violent or voluble a response to their overweight as this very heavy woman did. But most people with a weight problem are accustomed to being criticized, being laughed at, being psychoanalyzed by friends, family, employers, and strangers. All this weightism adds power to the pro-thin forces in society.

## YOUR OWN WORST ENEMY?

Cultural conditioning helps make the overweight person despise himself, so much so that the overweight person in this society can easily become his own enemy. He views his heaviness with embarrassment or shame. And these negative attitudes feed his guilt—make him feel guilty for the way he looks and the way he eats. This evolves into a general lack of self-esteem and self-confidence. Eventually, the result is self-hate. As the old cliché goes, "Nobody loves a fat man." And nobody does—not even the fat man himself. As earlier chapters emphasized, self-acceptance and self-respect are needed. But the prevalence of weightism does make maintaining self-esteem and a positive self-image inordinately hard for the overweight person.

These weightist attitudes about overweight aren't built into the human condition. They are simply a set of prejudices for this society in this era. Not every contemporary society is so virulently bigoted against the overweight. Contrast the American/Western European attitudes toward overweight to the commonly held beliefs of today's Russians. Overweight is no disgrace in Russia. There's an old Russian saying, still in common use, that translates roughly, "Abundance is kindliness, and kindliness is a good person. And the more there is of a good person, the better."

## GETTING BEYOND EXTERNAL APPEARANCES

Besides showing a benevolent attitude toward the overweight, that Russian saying brings up another important but often neglected point: the potential goodness of the human being who inhabits that "overweight" body. In this society, people associate self-worth and the worth of others with how they look—not how they feel, think, or act. Externals are considered of supreme importance, but internal factors are slighted or disregarded completely when judging a new acquaintance. Just one glance and you can pretty well categorize a person.

But is this categorization a fair one? We tend to glorify the package and ignore its contents. Is that thin, pretty woman sweet-natured and intelligent or shrewish and dumb? You can't tell until you talk to her, until you investigate beneath her surface beauty.

"Beauty's only skin deep," goes one proverb. But in this

society, we almost never look beneath the skin. Inner qualities like kindness, compassion, good humor, loyalty, and honesty make for a beautiful person just as surely as do slenderness and well-molded features.

But getting to know someone's inner qualities is too much trouble most of the time. Appearances must suffice all too often when we're in a crowd of strangers, whether on a busy city street, at a singles bar, at a football game, or at a party.

## RAISE YOUR CONSCIOUSNESS ABOUT WEIGHTISM

Now that you're aware of how weightist prejudice operates against the overweight, you have to make some important changes in your thinking regarding people's "packaging." You must continue to raise your consciousness about the cruelty and harm that weightism can foster. Now you have to *act* on the basis of your raised consciousness as well.

● First, you must make a conscious effort to separate your feelings about yourself, your appearance, and your self-worth from the mass of weightist prejudice and discrimination that you may face each day as a person with a weight problem.

If your overweight is slight—say, ten or fifteen pounds—this prejudice and discrimination may exist only in your own mind or in your competition for marriage and sex partners, for instance. If you are more noticeably overweight —say, thirty pounds or more—you may face much more painful and severe bigotry from thin, average-weight, and even fat people.

● Realize that these people are treating you in a bigoted, irrational manner when they make fun of your size or criticize your shape or give you problems in advancing on the job.

● Realize that you're dealing with ignorant, prejudiced people.

● Realize that their opinions are distorted by weightism.

- Realize that you are a worthwhile person, no matter how much weightism you may be subjected to.

- The important lesson to be learned in raising your consciousness about weightism is this: do not become your own enemy. That is, do not unthinkingly adopt the prejudices of the society around you toward the overweight.

Do not dislike yourself for what you are. Don't identify with the weightist "oppressor class" and turn against yourself and others like you.

It's important to have at least one friend you can always rely on—yourself.

## COMBATING WEIGHTISM

It's not enough merely to raise your consciousness about the existence of weightism, though that's a vital first step. Now you have to *do* something to change those patterns of prejudice. This isn't just "the right thing to do." This is a matter of self-preservation.

Just as you must learn not to adopt society's weightism and turn against yourself, you must learn not to turn against other overweight people. You must remind yourself constantly to look beyond the external packaging of people and appreciate their inner worth. Of course, you can't start a deep, probing dialogue with every person you meet on the street. Yet you can begin to fight weightism by eliminating it within yourself. You can begin to fight weightism by refusing to be an unconscious weightist yourself.

Let's say you see a woman walking down a supermarket aisle. She is a good forty pounds overweight and bulges unflatteringly out of too-tight polyester stretch pants. Don't allow yourself to make a disparaging remark to your companion about this woman's overweight. Don't even allow yourself to think that the woman "looks like a fat slob."

If the woman were a very dark-skinned black, for instance, you wouldn't think to yourself, "That woman is too black." You wouldn't say to your companion, "Boy, is that woman black!" as a means of ridiculing the woman, of putting her down behind her back. You would accept that woman's blackness as an integral part of her being.

Just the same, you must learn to accept other people's weight—heaviness or thinness—not as something good or bad in itself, but as something which makes each person a unique individual.

Don't think, "This person is too heavy." Just think, "This man or woman is a person, a unique person unlike anyone else." And it's great we can all look like ourselves, instead of looking like cardboard, conformist imitations of each other. Not everyone can be thin. Not everyone *should* be thin. We should all look the way we feel best, the way we are built to be, not the way weightist prejudice tells us we *should* look.

If you alone stop thinking prejudiced, unkind thoughts about other overweight people, you're not going to change the world. Weightism will not evaporate overnight. But you *will* eventually stop believing that there's only *one* "right" way to look. You *will* start feeling better about yourself, too, because you won't lump yourself into a group of people—overweight people—for whom you feel contempt or disgust or aversion.

Dropping weightism takes a big, uncomfortable weight off your shoulders—and off your mind.

You should also begin to raise the consciousness of your family, friends, and co-workers about weightism. You can make them aware that the overweight are treated like second-class citizens, that they are often made unwilling social outcasts. You can show your family and friends that weightism is just as unacceptable as prejudice toward any other minority group, such as blacks, orientals, Hispanics, women, and the aged.

And if you convince enough people to stop acting bigoted against the overweight—or to at least feel some guilt for their unacceptable bigotry—then you're going to help make your own life and the lives of millions of other overweight Americans easier and more pleasant. Because the problem of overweight isn't just going to go away miraculously.

We're not likely to find a vaccine against fat. We're not likely to find a permanent cure for obesity soon. But we can substantially diminish weightism in our lifetimes. And we can console ourselves with the flippant—but very true—saying: Thin may be in, but fat is where it's at.

It's a start.

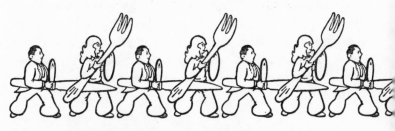

# 19 What's More Important than Being Thin?

Many things are more important than being thin. First and foremost, living fully and productively is far more important than the Pursuit of Thin. The quality of your life, of your day-to-day living, far outweighs the success or failure you might encounter in trying to become or stay thin.

Your life shouldn't be merely a succession of diets, a treadmill of fighting off fat attacks and atoning for the twin "sins" of overeating and midriff bulge.

Maybe you'll never be a *Vogue* model with cavernous cheeks and toothpick thighs. Maybe you'll never be as thin as a long-distance runner with a concave, hard-muscled stomach and protruding kneecaps. These just may not be realistic goals for you, based on your own understanding of your social and cultural environment, your psychological background, and your genetic makeup. But, as an earlier chapter amplified, you *can* be the best possible you.

Even if you're not at your "ideal" weight, you can have a strong, healthy, vibrantly attractive body. And you can appreciate yourself for your many good qualities—the notable attributes you listed on your personal assets inventory in Chapter 16.

You must appreciate your worth as a person, apart from

your compulsive/emotional eating, binges, diets, and what the scales might say.

What's more important than being thin? Living your life —*now*! Stop postponing your life until that mythical day when you will finally be "thin again" or "thin enough." Savor each day and live it to the fullest. Grab life boldly and squeeze all the pleasures and experiences you can from it. Think this way today, *act* this way today—and every day. Remember, today will never be repeated in your lifetime. So don't waste it.

Too many people with weight problems let their weight become a living problem, too. Compulsive/emotional eaters and overweight people tend to feel that they are less intrinsically important than thin people are. They put themselves down and diminish the potential quality of their lives.

What's more important than being thin? The feeling that you have a God-given *right* to a satisfying, happy life *right now*. You don't have to wait until you're thin or thinner to have the right to participate fully in the world as a first-class citizen.

Most overweight people feel that they're second-class citizens. This leads them to feel that they can't say no to other people's demands, especially if those other people are slim. Too often, people of substantial size feel they have to take care of a thin person's needs before taking care of themselves. The overweight person swallows the weightist prejudices that make him feel he should be ashamed of himself. So the heavier person may want to hide all the time, avoid social contact, become a kind of obesity dropout —all because he's terribly ashamed of his body and hence of himself.

All too often overweight people feel they are living or socializing on thin people's sufferance. The heavier people frequently feel they must be grateful that their lovers and spouses put up with their "disgusting, overeating" selves. This immediately places a relationship on a bad footing, if it doesn't poison the relationship altogether.

If you've read this far, you will recognize that the above attitudes and feelings of overweight, overeating people are counterproductive. These negative feelings are both useless and harmful. You can't allow yourself to fall into these ways of thinking. Nor can you allow weightist people to push you into feeling that way about yourself.

So what's more important than being thin? To stop putting yourself down and start building yourself up in your own estimation.

You're not going to swallow weightist prejudices anymore. And you're not going to think of yourself as a second-class citizen or as an inferior person, just because you have some extra pounds on you.

One good way to feel better about yourself and to tackle life with verve and vigor is to fight back. Yes, fight back against weightism directed at yourself and others. Become a kind of anti-weightism activist. This form of activism will daily convince you that it's correct to be proud of yourself and that anyone who tries to make you feel ashamed or inferior because of your weight is a bigoted fool.

What's more important than being thin? Getting rid of your fixation on the Pursuit of Thin.

Is thinking about being thin, planning how to get thin, worrying about not being thin, a good way to spend your time? Aren't there better, more creative, more emotionally nourishing ways to spend your day and to spend your life?

For tens of millions of people, the cream of their ingenuity and concentration is expended on the endless Pursuit of Thin. Do you *really* want to be like the skinny but diet-obsessed housewife who told us, "I myself lost fifty pounds and have kept it off for nine years. It hasn't been easy! You just have to decide that being thin is the most important thing in your life."

Is thinness worth being "the most important thing in your life"? Can't you think of some better things to do with your time, energy, and creative juices than focusing them so intensively on the perpetual Pursuit of Thin?

• • •

The fixation on getting thin wastes untold amounts of valuable, productive energies. Think of all the great achievers in world history who might not have achieved so much if they had been obsessed with dieting, eating, and the Pursuit of Thin.

If Shakespeare had been worried about keeping on his diet, he might not have had the time and energy to write *Hamlet, King Lear,* and *Othello.*

If Beethoven had been fixated on the Pursuit of Thin, he might have finished only *one* symphony, instead of nine.

If Michelangelo had been concerned about getting flabby thighs, the Sistine Chapel might today have a plain white ceiling.

If Benjamin Franklin had been obsessed with deflating his rotundity, there might have been no Franklin stove, no *Poor Richard's Almanack,* no bifocals, and no Declaration of Independence.

If Frank Lloyd Wright had spent his best hours away from his drafting board, thinking about how to reduce his waistline, instead of dozens of buildings there'd be dozens of holes in the ground today with brass markers: "Frank Lloyd Wright designed this hole."

If Catherine the Great had been obsessed with sticking to her diet, she might have wound up as Empress of Half the Russias, not All the Russias.

If Alfred Hitchcock had worried about his abdomen resembling a globe of the world, he might not have had the strength left to direct *The Lady Vanishes, North by Northwest,* and *Psycho.*

If Thomas Alva Edison had spent his time fretting about being twenty pounds overweight and paunchy, the world today might be without phonographs, motion-picture cameras, and light bulbs.

If Winston Churchill had spent his best years of "blood, sweat, and tears" working off his excess avoirdupois at a fat farm, today the British national anthem might be "Deutschland über Alles."

· · ·

You see how much world history could have been affected if great people had expended their valuable emotional, mental, and physical energies on the obsessive Pursuit of Thin? The world would be infinitely diminished.

Taking that down to a personal level, how much has your life been diminished by your preoccupation with getting thin, staying thin, and getting thinner? Surely, you have better things to do with your time and your brain than continually worrying about your weight!

If you hadn't been worried about going on a diet, breaking a diet, or staying on a diet, you might have taken up painting or photography. You might have taken up auto body mechanics or macramé. You might have started your own business or run for public office. You might have had a lot of happy, productive, creative times in your life—if only you hadn't been so fixated on the Pursuit of Thin.

Make up your mind now—you're not going to waste all those valuable years left in your life with an obsessive quest for thinness. You have more important things to do. *Use* your talents—or you'll waste them.

What's more important than being thin? Living up to your full potential—no matter how much you weigh.

Don't let overweight become a crutch, an excuse for not achieving your utmost potential.

Don't let overweight become a handicap, a reason for feeling crippled psychologically, physically, or socially.

And most of all, don't let overweight and overeating detract from the true business of your life—making your dreams come true.

What's more important than being thin? Enjoying a life lived to its full potential.

What's more important than being thin? Discovering the ultimate way to win out over the prejudiced skinnies of this world. For the compulsive/emotional eater, for the person who has spent the better part of a lifetime in the futile Pursuit of Thin, living happily is the best revenge.

What's more important than being thin? Liking yourself—just the way you are.

# Index